Healing the Emotions

DAN G. BLAZER, II, M.D.

D1295724

BROADMAN PRESS
Nashville, Tennessee

4269–26
ISBN: 0–8054–6926–5

Dewey Decimal Classification: 152.4
Subject heading: EMOTIONS

Library of Congress Catalog Card Number: 78–72278
Printed in the United States of America.

CONTENTS

Introduction

1. Man and His Problems   11
  The Nature of Man
  Psychological Problems
  Spiritual Problems

2. The Healing Resources of God   33
  God Provides His Word and His Spirit
  God Works Through Others to Heal
  Medicines and Specialized Environments for
    Healing

3. Seeking Help for Emotional Problems   45
  Pray to God About the Problem
  Talk with Someone You Trust
  Seek Professional Help, If Necessary
  Qualities of a Competent Therapist

4. The Role of the Spiritual Community   79
  Identify Capable Mental Health Workers
  Establish Relationships with Mental Health Workers
  Develop an Atmosphere of Support
  Establish a Prayer Ministry
  Develop Effective Counselors Within the Christian
    Community
  Conclusion

Notes   103

Reading List   105

HEALING THE EMOTIONS

INTRODUCTION

"Doctor, are you a Christian? I am not sure that I believe in psychiatry, but I must find some help. I sometimes wonder if I am emotionally disturbed." As a Christian and practicing psychiatrist I frequently hear a plea similar to the one stated above. Christians are finding themselves beset by problems on many different fronts that continually affect their sense of emotional well-being. Where does one go for help? How does one obtain help? Should a Christian seek professional or nonprofessional help? The purpose of this book is to answer some of these questions for my brothers and sisters in Christ. I hope that the material presented will serve as a liaison between Christians and the mental health professions.

The Christian inherently experiences some conflict when he attempts to adopt the teachings of Christianity and modern psychiatry. A major reason for this conflict is a confusion of roles. When one is experiencing anxiety or depression, it appears that assurances of relief come pouring forth from all corners.

The promises made by countless books on popular psychology sold in every book store sound so similar to the rest and peace promised by Christ that one naturally becomes bewildered.

The distinction between psychiatry and religion, however, has not always been so clouded. For years, the psychiatrist cared for the "insane" and "feeble-minded," while ministers and other church leaders cared for the emotional well-being of the populace at large. Increased secularization of society, changes within the church itself, and the advent of the modern psychotherapies have produced a profound change in this former division of labors. Psychiatry has taken over many functions of religion.[1] Therapy groups, encounter groups, and sensitivity groups have in many instances replaced the church as the setting of social and emotional interaction. Weekly, biweekly, and triweekly pilgrimages to the church have often been replaced by visits to the community mental health center or a private therapist's office. Psychiatry has also become more involved in the definition of values, long a function of religion. For example, alcoholism and compulsive gambling are now called "mental illnesses" and, for the former, treatment rather than admonishment or punishment is the normal recourse when such behavior is encountered.

Many churches, in contrast, have undertaken counseling programs such as marriage and family counseling that are kept operationally separate from the evangelical activities of the church. Little effort,

however, has been made to form a working alliance
between the church and psychiatry. In fact, many
feel that the Christian should not in any way be associated with the new psychiatry.[2] According to this
viewpoint, those truly "competent to counsel" are
Christians, and Christians alone. The profession of
psychiatry is not considered compatible with Christianity and is therefore regarded as an enemy. On
the other hand, psychiatry and religion have combined in an "unholy alliance" in which the Christian
faith is relegated to an inferior and ineffectual position. For instance, certain pastoral counselors conspic-
uously avoid discussing matters of faith in their sessions with clients.

As a Christian and a psychiatrist, I cannot accept
either of the above positions. God has given us, first
and foremost, redemption through his Son as stated
in his holy Word, the Bible. The spiritual life of man
must be considered and nourished in any therapy of
the whole person. Peter, however, encouraged us to
"supplement your faith with virtue, and virtue with
knowledge" (2 Pet. 1:5). The writer of Proverbs de-
clares that "wisdom abides in the mind of a man of
understanding" (14:33). We have gained, through the
years, an understanding of the thought processes,
emotions, and behavior of human beings. If we Christians are to be wise, we must not ignore this knowledge any more than we would ignore the need of
an appendectomy in an individual with acute appendi-
citis. I hope that this book will help Christians use

the knowledge and teachings accumulated by mental health workers over the years. At the same time, increased knowledge should help Christians guard against the pitfalls and weaknesses of modern psychological counseling and therapy. (The terms *psychotherapy* and *counseling* are used interchangeably in this book.)

Before we can explore what types of help are available for mental illness, it will be necessary to discuss the nature of mental illness. Emotional and mental anguish are not simple problems to understand, so bear with me as I attempt to clarify an often confused area.

1

MAN AND HIS PROBLEMS

Since the fall of man, we have been beset with the problems of living on earth. This is the state of mankind; every man and woman has a combination of physical, spiritual, psychological, social, and economic problems that interact with one another continually. Fifteen to twenty percent of the population of the United States have emotional difficulties (ranging from alcoholism to schizophrenia) that significantly interfere with their daily functioning. These individuals have been designated by most workers in the field as having "mental illness," though this is a woefully inadequate term. Regardless, clinical psychiatry is a specialized branch of medicine that deals with the study and treatment of these problems. This is only the tip of the iceberg however. In one study,[3] 65–75 percent of the residents of a Canadian community were "unhappy" and "dissatisfied" with their lives. If we are really honest with ourselves, most of us are not at peace with the world and with ourselves, not to mention our alienation from our Maker. Conflict, strife, inner turmoil, malaise, disinterest, and "lack of get up and go" are feelings com-

11

mon to each of us. Problems of living and unhappiness cannot be equated with mental illness, but they do remind us of the reality of some emotional disturbance in man and the potential for mental illness in each of us. How many of us have wondered, at least once, whether we were "going crazy" or whether we might be on the verge of a "nervous breakdown"? Mental illness is a real problem faced by those without and within the church and will, at some point, touch the lives of each of us, either directly or indirectly. Salvation does not guarantee a life free of psychological problems, and we would be remiss if we overlooked mental illness in Christians.

Problems of living are not new to our generation. As Job stated so well, "affliction does not come from the dust, nor does trouble sprout from the ground; but man is born to trouble" (Job 5:6–7). The writer of Ecclesiastes spoke in a similar vein. "For all his days are full of pain, and his work is a vexation; even in the night his mind does not rest" (Eccl. 2:23). Modern epidemiological studies have therefore verified what the Scriptures have taught for centuries. Yet how are we to understand and unravel the complexities of the problems of living?

Paul said, "May your spirit and soul and body be kept sound" (1 Thess. 5:23). Peter, in 1 Peter 3:8 said, "Finally . . . have . . . a tender heart and a humble mind." Within these two brief passages we find five separate terms that, in some way, describe the components of the spiritual and psychological nature of man. Before one can understand the problems besetting man, it is important to have some understanding of the nature of man.

There has been a struggle for years to appreciate the ultimate realities of the mind. We truly "see in a mirror dimly" (1 Cor. 13:12). It is probably fruitless to spend long hours in philosophizing about the nature of man, yet we must have some framework if we are to consider appropriate interventions to correct the problems besetting man. Rather than diagram and philosophize, let us first identify what we know to be the functional psychological and spiritual components of man.

The Nature of Man

A. The Soul

The Scriptures use the word *soul* to describe that part of man that survives death (Matt. 10:28). It is nonmaterial, given by God uniquely to man, and surely is the seat of his self-image, value system, strivings, and concepts of the meaning of life. It yearns to be united with God (Ps. 63:1; 84:2) but at the same time maintains free will (John 1:13; Gen. 3). The soul is the seat of the spirit of man (if spirit and soul can be divided).

For many years it was thought that the soul resided in the heart, but now most of us believe that it operates as a functional unit in close relationship with the brain or the nervous system. For Christians, the soul is as real as any part of our body or mind. Its nonmaterial nature in no way lessens its reality.

B. The Nervous System

The nervous system is something that we can see if we perform an autopsy on an individual's body after death. From our medical studies, we know the nervous system is material, subject to death and decay, and capable of many flaws in its performance. Examples of malfunctioning of the nervous system are the conditions of mental retardation and senility.

The nervous system is made up of the brain, the spinal cord, and the nerves of the body. In many ways it serves as a computer in that it receives information from the environment, processes that information, and produces output in the form of behavior. The physical transmission of information within the nervous system resembles quite closely the transmission of electrical impulses within a computer.

Certain parts of the nervous system are known to be involved with selective functions. For example, if an individual touches a hot stove, nerve impulses are carried up the nerves of the hand into the spinal cord where they connect with other nerves that leave the spinal cord and return to the muscles of the hand and arm. These nerves cause the individual to remove his hand very quickly from the stove. This is called a simple reflex. Therefore, the function of removing parts of the body from hot objects can be isolated and identified very easily within a certain portion of the nervous system. Yet there are many functions of the nervous system that cannot be isolated so easily within one or more than one parts of the brain, the spinal cord, or the nerves. Therefore we will consider the *functions* of the nervous system rather than trying to isolate where each of these functions can be located within the structure of the brain, spinal cord, or nerves.

The nervous system has a number of functional components, each of which can function quite adequately or be subject to illness or injury. They include the following.

Sensation. Sensation is the way in which an individual receives information from the environment. The five senses are vision, hearing, smell, taste, and touch. An individual can have a malfunction in one or more of these senses which may lead in turn to blindness, deafness, and so forth.

Perception. Perception is the ability to recognize a particular sensation that is received by the nervous system. For example, an individual who has damage to the back part of the brain may be able to see an object but may not be able to understand and appreciate what that object is. This medical condition is called "visual agnosia." The sensations of hearing, smell, taste, and touch may also not be "perceived" with injuries to other parts of the brain.

Cognitive Functioning. Cognition (or thinking) is the ability to process and integrate information from the environment, to solve problems, to reason, and to determine appropriate actions to be taken. Intelligence, abstraction, and mental capacity usually relate to cognitive functioning. Cognitive functioning can be disturbed in illnesses such as mental retardation or schizophrenia.

Emotion. Emotion is a complicated function that basically involves the mood or affect of an individual at a given point in time. The emotion of an individual may be depressed, anxious, elated, angry, apathetic, and so on. We have learned that a certain portion of the brain (the limbic system) is responsible for the emotional tone of an individual.

Emotion in many ways is a physiologic response to events that occur within the environment. An example of an emotional response would be the state of an individual who suddenly realizes that he has lost something of great value (such as his spouse). The emotional response might include a decreased appetite, inability to sleep, a depressed mood, a lack of energy, an inability to concentrate on events within the environment, and feelings of helplessness and hopelessness. Feelings are the cognitive representations of the emotions. For example, the emotional reaction described above would lead one to express feelings such as sadness and helplessness. An example of an illness that effects the emotions is manic depressive illness. In this condition, an individual has wide swings in the emotions (from extreme elation to deep depression) that seem to have very little relationship to events that are occurring within the environment of the individual.

Memory. The function of memory is the storage of information within the nervous system that is not immediately present in conscious thought but which is available for recall when necessary. Certain memories are very readily accessible (such as the memory of one's telephone number or address). Other memories are somewhat more difficult to recall but can be recalled after a period of time (such as the name of an old friend or the first line of a poem memorized in high school). Other memories are very difficult to recall and may be only available through certain special techniques (such as hypnosis). During hypnosis, memories of early childhood (before the age of five) may be brought to consciousness that were not available to conscious thought previously.

An example of a malfunction in memory is senility or organic brain disease. In this condition, an individual has great difficulty in remembering names, places, etc. Memory for events in the distant past may be relatively unaffected but the memory of events that have recently occurred may be very poor.

Drives (motivation). Every individual has basic drives to attain food, water, warmth, and sexual interaction. These are what I consider the lower order drives. They originate within the nervous system but may be felt within other parts of the body. For example, the drive to eat originates within a part of the brain called the hypothalamus but is felt within the body as a cramping and hyperactivity of the stomach. The drives lead an individual to alleviate the tension produced by these drives by appropriate behavior.

In the case of the drive to eat, the individual, by eating, satisfies the need created by the drive.

Injuries to the nervous system can cause problems with the drives. For example, an injury to a certain part of the hypothalamus can eliminate the drive to eat and an individual will literally starve to death because he will have no desire to eat. Similar problems can occur with the other drives as well.

Though modern psychology has said very little about them, there are very definitely higher order drives (or strivings) in addition to the lower order drives. I believe that these drives reside within the soul and consist basically of a desire to be united with God and interact socially with others. These strivings can certainly override the lower order drives and are therefore of more importance to the Christian. However, the lower order drives should not be neglected when one considers the nature of man.

The Activating System. Our body, in some ways, acts as a biological clock. We regularly spend periods of time asleep and awake. The typical pattern for most of us is that we sleep eight of every twenty-four hours. It is the activating system that informs us that we need sleep and in turn leads us to seek rest and sleep. In like manner, the activating system awakes us after we have attained a sufficient amount of sleep.

Malfunctions of the activating system lead to illnesses as well. One very interesting condition is that called narcolepsy. The individual suffering from narcolepsy may fall asleep at any given time during the day for ten or fifteen minutes. He seems to have no control over this behavior, and it thus can become very disturbing to him. An even more profound malfunction is that of coma in which the activating system is severely disturbed and an individual cannot be awakened from a very deep sleep.

As mentioned above, some of these functions of the nervous system can be isolated in certain structures within the brain but most are not so easily isolated and involve wide areas of the brain. Yet from our understanding of the performance of the nervous system, we know that physical problems within the body can lead to malfunction in each of the above seven functional components. For example, if the heart is not pumping enough blood to the brain, the individual will have difficulties in thinking (cognition) and memory (a condition we call delirium).

Problems in one functional component of the nervous system can lead to problems in other functions. A disease of the emotions, such as severe depression, can lead to a slowing of the thought processes, decreased memory, a poor self-concept, and even a change in the value system (such as a loss of hope of anything working out for the best).

Behavior. The nervous system expresses itself by behavior. This behavior may include such things as speech, action (such as walking, riding, sitting), or even activity. We, on the outside, looking at another individual can only gain some appreciation of the function of their soul and their nervous system by the behavior of that individual.

We have now seen that there are two realities that must be considered when one is trying to understand the nature of man. These realities are the soul and the nervous system. How do these two entities interact? Though no one has the ultimate answer to this question, the soul must in some way exist in a type of dynamic interaction with the nervous system. It affects the system and in turn is affected by it. As mentioned above, we (on the outside) can only "see" the soul through the behavior of another individual. Only God can see the soul clearly.

The division of the nature of man into the soul and nervous system and the further division of the nervous system into the seven functional components mentioned above are only divisions of convenience. Naturally, each of these components works in interaction with the other and in practice it is very difficult to make distinctions between each of these functions. In like manner, for the purposes of our further discussion, we will try to unravel and understand the complexities of the problems of living by separating spiritual from psychological problems. Again, such a classification is for our convenience, for the problems of living in man do not exist in isolation but interact with one another continually. Certainly the classification of these problems will have implications for whatever type of intervention is required to effect healing or relief from suffering. Carl Menninger, the well-known American psychiatrist, has stated, "It does little good to repent a symptom (a psychological problem), but it may do great harm not to repent a sin (a spiritual problem). Vice versa it does little good to merely psychoanalyze a sin, and sometimes great harm to ignore a symptom." Therefore let us consider the different types of psychological and spiritual problems that plague mankind.

Psychological Problems

Physical Conditions

Nowhere in the Scriptures are psychological problems which are caused by a physical condition more graphically presented than in Ecclesiastes 12.

"Remember also your Creator in the days of your youth, before the evil days come and the years draw nigh [old age], when you will say, 'I have no pleasure in them'; before the sun and the light, and the moon, and the stars are darkened [decreased vision in old age] and the clouds return after the rain [diminished intellectual powers]; . . . and one rises up at the voice of a bird [poor sleep and early awakening], . . . and terrors are in the way [suspiciousness and anxiety]" (vv. 1–2, 4–5).

The infirmities of old age are but one example of psychological problems that are related to physical illness and debilitation or physical abnormalities. A malfunction of the thyroid gland (called hyperthyroidism) in which a greater amount of thyroid hormone is produced than is needed by the body leads to nervousness, tremors, tension, a feeling of panic, and sweaty palms. We all experience similar symptoms when we walk down a dark, unknown street at night, but in this case the condition is produced by our fear of the unknown rather than a malfunction of the thyroid gland.

A tumor of the adrenal gland can cause one to become severely depressed, with lack of energy, poor sleep, and feelings that life is not worth living. The very same symptoms may develop in a person grieving the loss of a close relative or friend (in this case the adrenal gland is functioning normally). There is evidence that schizophrenia and manic-depressive illness are both caused (at least in part) by a biochemical abnormality in the brain. Further studies indicate that these two illnesses are inherited. One day we may discover what the abnormality is that causes schizophrenia and manic-depressive illness, just as we discovered that a deficiency of insulin is the cause of diabetes.

Certainly not all nor even most psychological problems are caused by physical problems, but this possible source of one's suffering must never be overlooked. Many unfortunate people have traveled from one counselor to another when they should have visited a physician for a physical checkup.

The Stresses of Life

As David was being pursued on all sides by King Saul and was in constant fear for his life, he cried out,

> Be gracious to me, O Lord, for I am in distress;
>> my eye is wasted from grief,
>> my soul and my body also.
> For my life is spent with sorrow,
>> and my years with sighing;
> my strength fails because of my misery,
>> and my bones waste away.
> I am the scorn of all my adversaries,
>> a horror to my neighbors,
> an object of dread to my acquaintances;
>> those who see me in the street flee from me.
> I have passed out of mind like one who is dead;
>> I have become like a broken vessel.
> Yea, I hear the whispering of many—
>> terror on every side!—
> as they scheme together against me,
>> as they plot to take my life. (Ps. 31:9–13).

A psychiatrist, and even someone without professional experience, who reads the above out of context must surely conclude that the writer is not mentally stable. Expressions of depression ("my eye is wasted from grief") and even paranoia ("I hear the whispering of many") pervade the entire passage. Yet David is experiencing what any human being would experience if placed under enough stress. We all have our

breaking points. Even at the points when all seems
lost, most people find ways of adapting that allow
them to maintain their sanity. David adapted in the
best way known; by casting his cares upon the Lord.
"But I trust in thee, O Lord,/I say, 'Thou art my
God.' My times are in thy hand;/deliver me from
the hand of my/enemies and persecutors!" (Ps. 31:14–
15).

Each of us may undergo psychological (grief),
social (a time of war), and economic (poverty) stress.
These stresses are known to affect the mental health
of those who are subjected to them. We have learned
to accept behavior from individuals grieving the loss
of a loved one (such as profuse crying, expressions
of hopelessness and despair, and an inability to function at work), that would not be tolerated under normal circumstances. However, we expect such behavior to resolve, over time, when the stresses have been
alleviated. Occasionally, however, individuals do not
recover their previous mental health when a stress
has been removed (such as in prolonged grief). These
stress situations may have brought to the surface previous problems that were never resolved.

Internal Conflict

Job declared that "My heart is in turmoil, and
is never still" (Job 30:27). Jesus pointed to the scribes
and Pharisees and said, "You are like whitewashed
tombs, which outwardly appear beautiful, but within
they are full of dead men's bones and all uncleanness,"

(Matt. 23:27). Our contradictory and conflictual nature is the cause of many of our difficulties. These conflicts can often be seen most clearly in young children, but they are present in each of us. For example, a young child may become very jealous when a new baby is born into the family. The child may fear that he will get less love and attention with the newborn around. Since children express their feelings so freely, it is not uncommon to hear such a child say, "I don't like my baby brother" or "I wish he would go away." Some children may even become physically abusive toward the new addition to the family. The older child soon learns, however, that his anger toward the newborn baby is not accepted by his parents. If he wishes his parents to love him, he must love the new baby. Thus a conflict between hating the baby and loving the baby develops. He is angry at the new baby for getting so much attention, yet he cannot express his anger for fear of disapproval from his parents. He also begins to feel true affection for the newborn. Normally, such conflicts are resolved as the child learns that his parents will continue to love him as well as the new baby, and he learns to love and care for his new sibling. Sometimes such conflicts are not resolved, but only covered over. They stay with us, even into adulthood. In the above example, if the conflict had not been resolved, the anger and hate toward the little brother could be covered over by an excess of concern for the little brother's safety and happiness. When the little brother receives a favor or praise, the old jealousy may be reawakened in the older sibling. This jealousy is often transformed into anxiety. The anxiety, in turn may persist as an anxiety reaction or be transformed into a symptom, such as compulsion (excessive handwashing) or a phobia (a fear of closed spaces). Each of us have internal conflicts that may place our heart in turmoil (anxiety). Underlying some of our good deeds are feelings of anger and jealousy (the dead men's bones within the whitewashed tombs). When such conflicts develop into symptoms, such as washing one's hands forty times a day, we call the illness a neurosis. Sigmund Freud contributed greatly to our knowledge of the conflictual nature of man (though there are many inadequacies and misconceptions in his writings).

Interpersonal Conflicts

As Paul and Barnabas were preparing for their second missionary journey, "there arose a sharp contention, so that they separated from each other; Barnabas took Mark with him" (Acts 15:39). Conflicts and contentions between people are just as prevalent today as they were in biblical times. Misunderstandings between friends and loved ones may cause much emotional suffering. We call such poor communications incompatibility, a generation gap, and games people play (the last designation being popularized in Eric Berne's book by the same name.[4] A "game" is an ongoing series of complementary, ulterior verbal "transactions" to a well-defined, predictable, but unhealthy outcome. Berne contends that such disordered communications result in much of the psychological pain that exists in our society). A piece of convincing evidence that a particular problem is an interpersonal problem is that there is often no problem when the other person is away.

Poor communication is seen nowhere better than in marriage conflicts. Two people who must live together, but who cannot communicate with one another, may find themselves most dissatisfied and discouraged with not only the marriage but with life in general. The marriage "counselor," who may be sought by a couple whose marriage is not working, seeks to accomplish one basic goal: the facilitation of better communication within the marriage. Once communication is improved, the marriage partners will often find themselves healthier and happier from a psychological standpoint.

Jesus recognized the fact that many problems exist because of poor communication or a lack of desire to communicate. He commanded us, "First be reconciled to your brother, and then come and offer your gift" (Matt. 5:24). "If your brother sins against you, go and tell him his fault, between you and him alone. If he listens to you, you have gained your brother" (Matt. 18:15).

Sin

"For out of the heart come evil thoughts, murder, adultery, fornication, theft, false witness, slander.

These are what defile a man" (Matt. 15:19–20). "Now
the works of the flesh are . . . enmity, strife, jealousy,
anger, selfishness, dissension" (Gal. 5:19–20). Sin continues to reign in this world. Even a well-known psychiatrist such as Karl Menninger is asking the question, "Whatever became of sin?" [5] We will discuss
sin in more detail in the following section. It is important, however, to emphasize that the fruits of sin may
be emotional problems. "Enmity," "strife," "anger,"
and "dissension" are not pleasant psychological states
and, in themselves, may lead a person to seek psychotherapy. Of course, in this instance, repentance
and a turning away from evil is the pathway to happiness and inner peace, not psychotherapy.

Spiritual Problems

The spiritual nature of man is as real as the physical and mental aspects of his being. God said, "Let
us make man in our image" (Gen. 1:26). Man, then,
was a companion of the Father, capable of admiring,
adoring, and enjoying God. He was unlike the remainder of creation, for he was an intellectual, moral, pure
and holy being.[6] In addition to his body, man has a
soul and a spirit. These are difficult concepts for the
philosopher, much less the scientist, to comprehend.
One cannot dissect the soul and spirit of man as one
can dissect a heart in a laboratory. One cannot explain
the work of the soul and spirit as one can explain
the behavior of a rat in a psychological experiment.
Nevertheless, we as Christians can attest to the reality

of our spiritual nature as readily as we can attest to the reality of the sun rising each morning.

Man, in addition, is a responsible being. Herein lies the spiritual problems of man. Let us consider these spiritual problems, especially as they relate to and may be confused with the psychological problems discussed above.

Alienation from God

Separation from the love of God is the underlying spiritual problem of mankind. "All men . . . are under the power of sin" (Rom. 3:9). This sin separates and alienates us from God's love. How do we become alienated from God? By our very nature, by the fact that we all are under the power of sin, we are alienated. How can the gulf between God and mankind be overcome? "They are justified by his grace as a gift, through the redemption which is in Christ Jesus" (Rom. 3:24). This justification is effected by our faith in Christ and our obedience to his will (Acts 2:37–38). Man may, through ignorance, continue in this state of alienation. These are the "lost sheep" mentioned in Matthew 10:6. They may not have true mental illness, but they often complain of a lack of direction, a lack of meaning to life and, interestingly, a "sense of alienation." Some may follow the psychotherapy route of joining encounter groups, undergoing an extensive psychoanalysis, or participating in sensitivity training. Others may become immersed in a social or political cause. Still others devote themselves to obtaining power and status. Others withdraw from society altogether (the members of communes and "drug freaks"). They rarely, however, attain happiness in any of these pursuits.

Most of these individuals function very well in whatever occupation they are pursuing and do reasonably well in their social and marital adjustment. Therefore they cannot be truly classified as having a mental illness. This does not mean that they enjoy their lives. They always sense that something is wrong.

Other individuals voluntarily and openly reject the love of God. These are those who "blaspheme against the Holy Spirit" (Mark 3:29) and the professed atheists. They take pride in their freedom from religion and attempt to fight anything that implies the existence of God. These individuals are not happy or satisfied with their existence and the overt anger they direct toward God covers a deeper need for the concern and care for a loving Father. Pride, however, separates them from his love, they rarely attain the peace they seek through their own efforts.

Living in Sin

Some profess a belief in God but blatantly live sinful lives. Paul described these individuals well:

"For although they knew God they did not honor him as God or give thanks to him. . . . Therefore God gave them up in the lusts of their hearts to impurity . . . to dishonorable passions . . . and receiving in their own persons the due penalty for their error. . . . They were filled with all manner of wickedness, evil. . . . Though they know God's decree that those who do such things deserve to die, they not only do them but approve those who practice them" (Rom. 1:21–32).

We see these people all around us. New York City has often been labeled "Sin City." If one walks down Forty-second Street, one quickly becomes aware of the depths to which man's manifest sinful acts have taken him.

Christians are occasionally disturbed when those participating in such sinful acts do not appear immediately to suffer adverse consequences. It is true that, at any given time, these individuals may not be suffering from any significant emotional problems (for example, the "well-adjusted" homosexual). These acts, however, ultimately lead to destruction, "For the wages of sin is death" (Rom. 6:23). For most, however, the "due penalty for their error" occurs during their lifetime (as happened with the prodigal son), and death is only the final defeat in a life that exists on the "skid rows" of society.

Demon Possession and Demon Influenced Individuals

"A man with an unclean spirit who lived among the tombs and no one could bind him any more, even with a chain. . . . Night and day among the tombs and on the mountains he was always crying out, and bruising himself with stones. . . . And Jesus asked him, 'What is your name?' He replied, 'My name is Legion; for we are many. . . . And the unclean spirits came out, and entered the swine" (Mark 5:2–13). During the time of Christ there can be no doubt that a major spiritual problem that could result in profound emotional disturbances was demon possession. Many contend that demon possession continues to be a major problem in modern society.[7] Others would argue vehemently against this proposition. All true Christians must agree, however, that Satan is alive and continues to tempt us and influence us for evil with every means available to him. We must ever be watchful, for "your adversary the devil prowls around like a roaring lion, seeking some one to devour" (1 Pet. 5:8).

In conclusion, let me again emphasize that the problems on this earth are seldom simple, neither are they easily categorized. The classification presented above is for our convenience. It would be unusual for an individual to have one of these problems in isolation. Psychological problems are rarely related to internal conflict alone, but usually involve real stress of life and problems of communication as well. In a parallel manner, the spiritual problem of alienation from God is almost always associated with sinful living (and you may be assured that the devil will have his hand in the matter). Psychological problems and spiritual problems usually exist, side by side in the same individual. One should not be emphasized in our treatment approaches to the exclusion of the other. This is treatment of the *whole person.*

2
THE HEALING RESOURCES OF GOD

"And God is able to provide you with every blessing in abundance, so that you may always have enough of everything" (2 Cor. 9:8). "Now to him who by the power at work within us is able to do far more abundantly than all that we ask or think" (Eph. 3:20). The Scriptures are replete with passages reminding us that for every problem we experience, God has provided solutions. The resources for healing available from God are many. Let us take a look at some of the resources available for emotional healing.

God Provides His Word and His Spirit

"Lo, I am with you always" (Matt. 28:20). "Happy is he who trusts in the Lord" (Prov. 16:20). "But the Counselor, the Holy Spirit, whom the Father will send in my name, he will teach you. . . . Peace I leave with you; . . . Let not your hearts be troubled, neither let them be afraid" (John 14:26–27). "Thy word is a lamp to my feet, and a light to my path" (Ps. 119:105). When trouble besets us, regardless of its origin, it is to God that we turn. Unfortunately, however, we often turn to God as a last resort rather than as an initial response. So often we may read of

a desperate soul when, having reached "the end of
the road," turns back to his Father, and is rescued
from the "miry clay" (such as the prodigal son). If
we could only keep our priorities straight, we could
save ourselves months and even years of distress. If
one makes a wrong turn in life or if one is oppressed
by stress from without, it is at the beginning of the
difficulty, not at the end, that he should turn to his
Maker. As we consider a pathway to recovery from
emotional illness, we must always place God first and
foremost in our plans.

God Works Through Others to Heal

"Every good endowment and every perfect gift
is from above" (Jas. 1:17). "For he that is not against
us is for us" (Mark 9:40). God has worked his will
through many great leaders in the past (Dan. 2:20–
21) and continues to do so today (Rom. 13:1). He sent
his angels to minister to the needs of Jesus in the
wilderness (Matt. 4:11). Surely he can work his will
through those in the helping professions (both Christian and non-Christian). We inherently believe this
when we pray that God "guide the hand of the sur-
geon." We can, with equal confidence in the power
of God, pray that he "guide the counselor and the
psychotherapist." Mental health professionals come
from various backgrounds with different types of
training and different orientations. Such professionals
may be called psychiatrists, clinical psychologists, social workers, pastoral counselors, marriage counse-

lors, and psychotherapists of various descriptions. We will discuss the qualifications and orientation of some of these professionals later. It is sufficient for the present to say that competent and genuinely caring individuals can be found in each of these specialties.

Let us look now at the psychosocial therapies. Paul and James have both indicated that there is a need to be integrated or single-minded in order for an individual to function properly (Col. 3:22; Jas. 1:7–8). Those not single-minded have difficulty with integration which in turn leads to problems in functioning (an obvious example is the conflict that Paul experienced in Rom. 7). The goal of psychotherapy and counseling is to achieve mental health. Mental health basically implies successful functioning. We might consider mental health as the ability to love (relate to others), to work effectively, and to be relatively free of conflict (being honest with one's self). I believe this is basically what Paul and James were talking about when they described the necessity of the Christian being single-minded in order to live a happy life and to work effectively.

The psychosocial therapies are poorly understood. It would serve us well to demythologize these therapies and try to understand the basic ingredients of successful psychotherapy and counseling.

What is psychotherapy? Jerome Frank has stated that, "Psychotherapy encompasses all those activities by which one person seeks to relieve the distress and beneficially affect the behavior of another through psychological means." In one way, all psychotherapy leads to integration which in turn leads to a change in behavior that is more constructive and more satisfying. Though in many ways the psychosocial therapies remain an art, experience in some scientific studies have lifted these therapies above the intuitive.

There are many different types of psychosocial therapies. These include psychoanalysis, individual therapy or counseling, marriage and family therapy, and group therapy. The goals of the psychosocial therapies, however, are generally fairly uniform. These goals include (1) *symptom removal* (such as a pain in the stomach that may be due to emotional problems), (2) *behavior change* (such as constructive behavior in a school setting as opposed to destructive behavior), (3) *insight* (gaining a greater understanding of the motivation of one's behavior which in turn would provide an individual with the ingredients necessary to lead to behavior change), (4) *improved social efficiency* (such as the ability to relate in a more adult manner with one's peers), and (5) *education* (increased knowledge of behaviors of others and how people typically interact).

Do the psychosocial therapies work and if so how? It appears that the conditions necessary for the psychosocial therapies to succeed are the following.[8]

A Shared World View

It is important that the therapist and the patient or client* agree on the nature of the world. Therefore, when a problem is identified (named) then the identification of the source of the problem can be accepted by both the therapist and the *patient* or *client* (these terms will be used interchangeably). In a primitive society, a particular problem may be identified as invasion by a spirit. If both the witch doctor and the individual who comes to the witch doctor for help agree that this is the cause of the individual's problem, the chances of gaining healing through the activities of the witch doctor are greatly enhanced. In the same manner, if a member of Western society seeks the help of a psychiatrist, it is important that both agree that the problem may be due to difficulties such as in interpersonal relationships or problems in one's childhood.

An Interpersonal Relationship Where the Therapist Shows an Accurate Empathy and a Nonpossessive Warmth and Genuineness in the Interaction. All of the psychosocial therapies are interpersonal relationships. The chances for success in therapy are greatly enhanced when the therapist is empathic and cares about the client or patient which he is treating. The therapist conveys to the patient, "I really want to know what you mean" or "I'd like to hear clearly what you are saying."

The Patient or Client Expects to Get Better. The therapist who does not believe that his techniques will be successful and who does not believe in himself will generally have very little success in treating the problems that are brought to him. If, on the other hand, the therapist emanates confidence in himself and in the patient, the patient has hope. This hope is of great value in leading to successful therapy.

Techniques Are Used That Are Relevant to One's World View

As mentioned above, gaining insight into one's behavior is a culturally accepted technique that is seen to be of value in alleviating the emotional distress of individuals in modern Western society. In like manner, praying together by two Christians is understood by Christians as being a very effective technique by which an individual might receive emotional healing.

The following processes take place in psychotherapeutic experiences to promote healing.

Confession. In almost every type of therapeutic experience in almost every culture, the process of confessing one's faults and receiving a sense of forgiveness (in the form of acceptance, understanding, or sense of being forgiven by one's Father in heaven) is an essential ingredient in leading to a change in one's behavioral and emotional state.

Learning. Learning can occur in a number of ways. For example, a patient can learn more acceptable ways in dealing with certain problems (such as anger) by imitating the behavior of the therapist who may be able to accept the anger of the patient. In addition, the patient may learn techniques of socialization in that the therapist may teach the individual new ways of dealing with life situations. He also may teach the patient new communication techniques. A third type of learning that can occur in the psychosocial therapies is a linkage of feelings and behavior. The individual may come to a counselor initially with behavior that is persistent but which is not well understood. The therapist, in turn, helps the patient to connect that behavior with feelings that the patient may not have been aware of. Once the patient has learned that certain feelings and behaviors are connected, he is in a better position to be able to change his behavior.

Possibly the most important type of learning that occurs in therapy, however, is that the patient learns to see himself differently. A basic goal of therapy is to help the patient attain a more positive view of himself (such as an improved self-image or increased self-esteem).

The Corrective Emotional Experience. If the patient in the psychosocial therapeutic experience sees that he is being understood, accepted, and dealt with honestly, this in itself may be a very important factor in the improvement of the individual. Poor experiences in relating to others in the past and poor experiences with significant individuals in the individual's life (such as parents who have not loved and cared for an individual correctly) can be greatly alleviated by a positive experience with another important individual. The importance of the corrective emotional experience should never be underestimated.

Some have called this process *reparenting.* Christians are well aware that each of us undergoes the therapeutic process of reparenting when we accept God as our Father when converted. Our experience with a perfect Father overcomes many of the previous bad experiences we had had with our natural parents.

God Provides Medicines and Specialized Environments for Healing

Medicines for Healing

The good Samaritan went to the man journeying from Jerusalem to Jericho "and bound up his wounds, pouring on oil and wine; . . . and brought him to an inn, and took care of him" (Luke 10:34). God has provided us today with many medications that are infinitely more effective than oil and wine. It is not by chance that some of our most potent drugs are natural products. Digitalis (the dried leaf of the common foxglove) is a powerful and effective stimulant of the heart. Insulin (the natural product of the human pancreas) is replaced artifically by injections in the diabetic. Lithium carbonate, a salt of one of the basic elements, is the most effective treatment of manic-depressive illness known. Many feel it works by, in some way, replacing a chemical that is depleted in the brain of the person with manic-depressive illness.

Though psychotropic (nerve) medications are frequently given indiscriminately by physicians and are abused by patients, there is no question that drugs like Chlorpromazine (Thorazine) have helped thousands of emotionally incapacitated individuals to return to a functional existence. Since the introduction of Thorazine in the early 1950s, the patient population of the state mental hospitals in this country has been cut in half (though the incidence of schizophrenia and other incapacitating illnesses has remained unchanged). We are continuing to develop new medications and to learn how to better use the medications that we have.

It is important to remember that most medications given for "nerves" (Valium, Librium, Triavil, Seconal) are *not* prescribed by psychiatrists but by other medical specialists. We in the psychiatric profession are continually trying to educate our other medical colleagues about the proper use of these drugs. Usually we suggest *less* rather than more use of such medicines. It is our responsibility as physicians to use these drugs effectively. I can honestly say that my psychiatric colleagues have made a concerted effort to use such drugs wisely and discriminately.

God has given us a great repertoire of balms for the emotionally disturbed. Alas, many physicians hand out drugs such as Valium as if it were candy. We, as Christians, should be wary of such indiscriminant prescriptions. One should ask his physician the *specific* reasons that any such medications is being prescribed. We, as consumers, are not obligated to take everything handed to us by a man in a white coat. At the same time, a general "fear of drugs" may deprive one of a beneficial remedy to a troublesome problem.

Effective medications have been developed for the treatment of schizophrenia, manic-depressive illness, severe depressive illness, acute panic attacks, bed-wetting, and hyperactivity in children. One word of caution is in order. Though there are medications that are effective sleeping pills for one or two nights, *no* sleeping pill is effective over an extended period of time. Anyone taking such a medication for over two to three weeks probably is experiencing more harm than good from the drug. The bottom line is that both doctor and patient must be wise and cautious when a psychotropic drug is being considered.

Environments for Healing

God also provides specialized environments for healing. As the inn served the good Samaritan as a place for healing to take place, the modern hospital serves in a similar capacity today. In fact, the word *hospital* comes from the Latin word *hospitale*, which means a house or institution for guests.

The care of the mentally ill in hospitals has gone through a number of phases. During the Dark Ages, the prescribed treatment for mental illness was torture and death. Philippe Pinel in 1793 ordered the chains removed from mental patients in Paris and ushered in a new era of treatment and humane concern. Still, until recent years, the major task of the state mental institution was the physical care and control of inmates. Now many techniques are available to us and the hospital milieu has become an integral part of the therapeutic experience (instead of being primarily custodial). Unfortunately, reforms have been slow secondary to acute personnel shortages, pyramidal systems of authority in the interest of efficiency, and lack of public interest and concern. Hospitalization is still necessary for the management of certain emotional states in both Christians and non-Christians. In fact, an individual who is acutely depressed to the point of suicide may literally have his life saved by a brief psychiatric hospitalization. Reforms in our mental institutions must continue, but we as Christians and as members of the general public must change many of our negative attitudes toward the psychiatric hospital.

Hospitalization can provide other very important services to the acutely and severely mentally ill individual. The relief from the external pressures of a very difficult environmental situation (such as taking a child out of a family where marriage conflict is rampant) may in itself be quite helpful in leading to improvement in an emotionally disturbed child. Hospitalization also may enable a severely disturbed individual to relearn socialization techniques in a controlled environment. As such, the same techniques that might be used with an individual as an outpatient who is less severely disturbed can be used within the hospital setting for the more disturbed. This is what has been commonly referred to as the *milieu*. It has proven to be a very effective means of helping certain types of individuals better cope with the world outside of the hospital setting.

Certain types of emergency psychiatric treatments can be instituted only within the hospital setting because of the necessity of proper control for such treatments. Many medications are best begun in a hospital and the response of an individual to that medication can therefore be evaluated.

In summary, hospitalization can be important and sometimes lifesaving in the total treatment approach to the emotionally disturbed. Its value should not be underestimated. Each of us has some responsibility for seeing that improved conditions within our psychiatric hospitals lead to more effective treatments.

3

SEEKING HELP FOR EMOTIONAL PROBLEMS

Help is available to the emotionally disturbed, but finding that help can be a difficult process. Here are certain steps that are generally applicable to finding help but first a word of caution. One must remember that any written material is at a distinct disadvantage. No two individual problems are alike and there is *no* "handbook" that will be totally satisfactory. Many books are written that promise peace and happiness if you follow certain steps. The Christian must beware of such empty promises. The best guidebook ever written for the emotionally disturbed is the Bible. All other literature must necessarily be used *only* to evoke prayerful consideration of different possibilities for healing.

Pray to God About the Problem

"Is there anyone among you suffering? Let him pray" (Jas. 5:13). We have countless illustrations of godly men and women in Old and New Testament times going to God in a time of need. These believers poured out their hearts to God for hours at a time, (as Jesus did in the garden of Gethsemane). If we look carefully at the process and progress of these prayers, we often find that encouragement comes even during the prayer itself. The weak and distressed David in Psalm 31:9 ("Be gracious to me, O Lord, for I am in distress") becomes the strong and encouraging David in the twenty-fourth verse of the same psalm ("Be strong, and let your heart take courage, all you who wait for the Lord!"). We all have had such experiences during fervent prayer, but how soon we forget.

I have found in my work with Christians that being honest with God about emotional problems is not an easy task. We tend to hide our own inadequacies from ourselves. Once a young woman came to me because her husband had deserted her. She had prayed for hours that God would help her to overcome her depression after this event. For months nothing changed and finally she sought professional help. I found that she was angry to the point of rage at her former husband, but she could not admit this to herself. Only when she could candidly say to herself and to God that her primary problem was anger did she pray that God would relieve her anger and forgive her. At that point, she could truly forgive her husband and the depression improved. Her prayers became effective when she prayed with "understanding" as well as with the "spirit" (1 Cor. 14:15).

One of Jesus' disciples asked him to teach them to pray (Luke 11:1). Paul told us that "we do not know how to pray as we ought, but the Spirit himself intercedes for us . . . . according to the will of God" (Rom. 8:26–27). When we first experience an emotional problem, we should not assume we understand the cause and pray for relief only. We should pray first for understanding and guidance in our actions to correct the problem, whether the proper behavior is to seek further help or to correct our own behavior. Our prayers then continually evolve over time, as our understanding of the problem improves.

Once we pray a fervent prayer, we must be willing to listen to God's answer. This involves being sensitive to doors that are open *and* doors that are closed forever. God is answering us every moment of the day, but we often have difficulty accepting his answers.

God is not only the starting point for effecting true healing. He is also the one source of strength upon which we can always rely. Micah, at a time when all about him were turning away from the Lord, said, "Put no trust in a neighbor, have no confidence in a friend; guard the doors of your mouth from her who lies in your bosom; for the son treats the father with contempt, ... But as for me, I will look to the Lord, I will wait for the God of my salvation, my God will hear me" (Micah 7:5–7). A great emotional crisis can arise when we see those around us turn away from God's truth. If friend, neighbor, and even spouse leave the Way, our spiritual journey may be very lonely and we may become quite discouraged. Yet God *never* fails us and will continually show his love to us. "Lo, I am with you always, to the close of the age" (Matt. 28:20).

Talk with Someone You Trust

"Bear one another's burdens" (Gal. 6:2). "Confess your sins to one another, and pray for one another that you may be healed" (Jas. 5:16). The Bible is very clear on one point. Do not keep your problems to yourself! Find someone you trust and talk about your problems with them. This person may be your spouse, a good friend, an elder, a minister, or a physician. There is much peace available in just verbalizing the difficulty. Tension may be relieved. The problem may not be as great as initially imagined.

Often the person that one should talk with initially is the person with whom one is having difficulty. "Therefore, putting away falsehood, let every one speak the truth with his neighbor" (Eph. 4:25). "If your brother sins against you, go and tell him his fault, between you and him alone. If he listens to you, you have gained your brother" (Matt. 18:15). If there is an admonition concerning interpersonal relations in the Scriptures, being direct and honest with our brother is that admonition. Unfortunately, we go at times to extreme ends to avoid direct confrontation.[9] In my own practice, I often serve as a sounding board for the difficulties one person is having with another. People come to me and literally work for hours in developing enough courage to speak to a spouse or parent about a matter of discord. Yet talking with the person, not a counselor, is the most quick and effective way of dealing with interpersonal conflicts.

Seek Professional Help, If Necessary

Services Available from the Mental Health Profession

The mental health profession can offer a number of services to the emotionally disturbed. Unfortunately, most people in the lay public believe that you go to a psychiatrist and position yourself on a couch for four or five years. This only occurs in a minority of instances. Psychotherapy continues to be the primary service that most mental health professionals offer, but psychotherapy takes many forms. Let us look at the relative benefits of the psychotherapies (without delving into individual schools of thought) and also consider other services that are available.

Psychotherapy and Counseling. Psychotherapy and counseling may include psychoanalysis, insight-oriented psychotherapy, group therapy, family therapy, and marriage counseling. Mental health workers have acquired a body of knowledge about emotional illness over the last few years that has led the practice of psychotherapy and counseling from a pure art form into a system that has a fair scientific base. Let us be honest about what we know however. Psychotherapy is an empirical science at best (a science that relies on experience or observation alone). Yet psychotherapy is effective in many, though not all, instances.

The approach of the consumer, patient, should be similar to that of Gamaliel (Acts 5:38–39) and Jesus (Matt. 7:16); namely, see if the results are worthwhile. Many Christians and non-Christians have, in fact, "tested the market" and today psychotherapy flourishes as never before, in spite of the frequent comments that psychiatry is in a crisis. All empirical sciences will be in a continual state of flux and crisis until exact systems and procedures are developed to guide the applied aspects of that science. We are far from such an understanding of human behavior. Many have equated our practice of psychotherapy today with the practice of medicine seventy-five years ago. The practice of medicine has changed dramatically over the past seventy-five years, but no one would question the value of medicine at the turn of the century in the overall care of those in ill health. Yet many medical practices at that time were more harmful than helpful. In the practice of the art of medicine, namely relating to the physically and mentally ill, the psychotherapist is generally more empathic and effective than his nonpsychiatric cohort.

The terms *counseling* and *psychotherapy* have been used interchangeably in this book. *Counseling* literally means to advise or recommend a course of action. *Psychotherapy* literally is the application of various forms of mental treatment to nervous and mental disorders. Certainly one component of most of the psychotherapies is to advise. The techniques of value in successful psychotherapy may, in like manner, be applied to successful counseling. Therefore, until we gain a greater understanding of the psychosocial therapies, arbitrary distinctions between counseling and psychotherapy per se are of little value. We would do better to describe the nature and techniques of the particular interactions in which we are engaged. For example, the techniques of psychoanalysis and client-centered therapy have been well described by Sigmund Freud and Carl Rogers respectively.

Evaluation Services. The causes of emotional disturbance are often quite complicated and may involve a combination of physical, psychological, social, and economic problems. Before any type of intervention is attempted to correct a particular difficulty, a thorough evaluation is in order. Evaluation services are critical in the management of emotional illness. Proper evaluation of an individual's problem should take into account physical, social, and economic as well as psychological factors. Many clinics take a multidimensional approach to diagnosis of mental illness. This is especially true for clinics that work with special age groups (child guidance clinics, developmental evaluation clinics, geriatric clinics) or with special problems (alcoholism or drug abuse). These clinics employ professionals from a number of disciplines (medicine, psychology, social work, and even law) who work together in an interdisciplinary team. Though these evaluation clinics often take many weeks to work up a given client, they are generally quite competent and professional in their approach to the troubled individual.

Psychotropic Medications. As mentioned above, specific medications have been developed for the treatment of a number of emotional illnesses (schizophrenia, manic-depressive illness). A well trained physician (usually a psychiatrist) is required to properly administer such medications.

Behavior Therapy. Though behavior therapy has received much adverse publicity in recent years, when used properly it can be a valuable tool for the mental health worker. For example, an obese individual can be taught to go through certain procedures at each meal (chewing each mouthful of food ten times before swallowing) that enable him to lose weight more effectively. In the opposite condition of anorexia nervosa (severe weight loss related to psychological problems) behavior therapy can literally be lifesaving.[10] In fact, we use behavior therapy every day. Whenever we discipline ourselves to work more efficiently or try to correct a bad habit, we use the principles of behavior therapy.

The Physical Therapies (Electroshock Therapy). The thought of shock therapy usually strikes fear into the heart of the layman. It is true that, at one time, it was used indiscriminately and was not a safe procedure. Today, however, the use of electroshock therapy is limited to the treatment of severe depressions (individuals who are often acutely suicidal). It is a completely painless procedure that is one of the safest treatments in medicine. Though there is some memory loss at the time of the treatment, memory almost always returns completely. Treatments, as they are given today, *do not* make a "zombie" out of the patient.

The Christian must again take a cautious but rational approach to this therapeutic form. Above all, we must not develop preconceived prejudices about acquaintances or fellow Christians who have undergone electroshock therapy. These prejudices may inhibit us from showing love and concern for such an individual, thereby causing more harm for the person than we imagined caused by the treatment itself.

The Christian Counselor

If it is agreed that professional help is necessary, how does the Christian identify a competent professional? One approach is to seek a Christian practitioner. David said in the Psalms, "The mouth of the righteous utters wisdom, and his tongue speaks justice" (Ps. 37:30). Adams (2) feels that *only* Christians are "competent to counsel" other Christians and bitterly attacks non-Christian mental health workers. Certain secular writers would agree to some extent. Torrey says that the best therapists for a given culture (the Christian way of life) are those who come from within that culture.[11] For example, it is very difficult for the non-Christian practitioner to understand the concept of grace. We Christians can accept the fact that we are all guilty in the sight of God (this is real

guilt, not neurotic guilt), but our guilt does not necessarily lead to a neurosis. For the man who has no
God, guilt is an unacceptable psychological state precisely because there is no readily available source of
relief from that guilt. The guilt is then "transformed"
into a neurotic symptom, such as a phobia, which is
a more acceptable psychological state. The Christian
can bypass this psychopathological condition by accepting the grace of God, namely the forgiveness of
sin through the death of Jesus (Rom. 8). It is true
that Christians develop neurotic symptoms because
of "unrealistic" guilt (guilt based on fantasy rather
than reality), and these guilty feelings can be alleviated by psychotherapy. Yet the Christian counselor
has the added advantage of being able to help the
Christian to overcome his "realistic" guilty feelings
(such as the continual sins of the flesh mentioned in
Rom. 7:13–24).

Secular psychotherapy has overstepped its rational boundaries precisely at this point. Freud correctly perceived that an individual could develop neurotic symptoms because of repressed guilty feelings.
Upon exploration of these feelings (which he called
psychoanalysis), his patients were able to remember
past events and the feelings associated with these
events were greatly diminished when the events became known to the conscious mind. He became so
enamored that he believed *all* guilt was of neurotic
origin and went so far as to postulate that religion
itself was the product of the need of the unconscious

mind to expiate itself of guilt. This was his fatal mistake. We, as Christians, can learn from the discoveries of Freud, but, as rational consumers of the knowledge available, do not have to accept those tenets of his theories that are contrary to our Christian beliefs.

Yet being a Christian does not imply competence in the area of counseling and psychotherapy. The Christian practitioner may be well-meaning but poorly trained and inexperienced. In particular, many Christian therapists are quite good at working with certain types of problems but do not know their own limitations. (It should be stated emphatically from the beginning that those problems I see in certain well-meaning but ineffective Christian counselors are no less a problem for any untrained, inexperienced counselor, regardless of orientation). A particular problem is alcoholism. Alcoholism is a complicated metabolic, psychological, and spiritual state. The minister or counselor who attempts to treat an alcoholic without support from other sources actually does his counselee a disservice. For example, abrupt withdrawal from alcohol may precipitate an agitated condition called delirium tremens or D.T.'s. If the condition is not handled by a physician, the alcoholic may develop seizures which can ultimately lead to death. In addition, alcoholism is a very lonely condition. There is excellent emotional and often spiritual support forthcoming from a group like Alcoholics Anonymous that the individual counselor cannot give. If these and other resources are used along with Christian therapy, the opportunity for success in working with this very difficult problem is greatly multiplied.

Untrained Christian therapists may also fall short of effective therapy in their inability to identify the problem of the counselee. A minister once asked me about a woman in his congregation who regularly came to him for help with a particular problem. She was having an affair of which her husband had no knowledge. She demanded the utmost confidentiality from the minister but hoped that he could help her to terminate the illicit relationship. The minister prayed with her frequently for forgiveness of her immorality, and she listened to his advice about how to rid herself of the other man and willingly received his chastisement for her sinful behavior. These visits went on for months, yet the affair continued. Finally the minister was desperate for advice. After discussing the situation at length, we both agreed that the "real" sin of this woman was her anger toward men. Through her behavior she continually "got back" at her husband by carrying on an affair behind his back. At the same time she put down the minister "covertly" by demonstrating how ineffective his therapy had been. Without being able to understand the motivation for her behavior, the minister played right into her persistent pattern. The woman's prayers and the prayers of the minister were ineffective because the real sin (her controlling and destructive behavior toward men) had not been identified. In some ways, this situation reminds one of the fairy tale "Rumplestilskin." The woman in this story could only over-come her problem with the little man when she could name him. "I will pray with the spirit and I will pray with the mind also" (1 Cor. 14:15). If our prayers for forgiveness and strength to change are to be effective, we must understand (name) the problem we are praying about.

A third problem with the well-meaning but un-trained and inexperienced therapist is that of the "hidden motive." One can generally feel confident of the motives of a true Christian who is a therapist; but this may not always be the case. One such hidden motive is the need to "preach" to those with problems. This interferes with the counselor's ability to actively listen to the counselee. Another common and poten-tially dangerous hidden motive that warrants special attention is as follows.

The therapist may be attracted to a pretty young woman who has marital problems. Though he con-sciously tries to encourage the woman to strengthen her marriage, he may unconsciously wish her to ad-mire him as a much more desirable and caring individ-ual than her husband. He then makes himself available to her at almost any hour and frequently "rescues" her from difficult situations. He goes out of his way to "take her side" when marital conflicts arise and praises her frequently. The woman then finds herself attracted to the counselor, misinterprets his conscious motives (though correctly interpreting his hidden mo-tives), and wishes to make more of the relationship than therapy. The situation may then escalate to one of embarrassment and guilt for both parties. During this process, the counselor loses his ability to counsel, and the marital problem is further complicated rather than improved. Training in counseling, under supervision, is the best way I know to avoid these pitfalls.

In conclusion, one must be wise in choosing a counselor. A Christian background may be a big plus in the selection process but does not guarantee competency in counseling. Just as there are many excellent Christian counselors and many poor and potentially dangerous secular counselors, there are ineffective and often damaging Christian counselors and properly motivated and competent secular counselors. But how does one select a competent counselor?

Qualities of a Competent Therapist

A Christian Therapist or a Therapist Who Is Not Antagonistic to Christianity

Most competent professionals are not atheistic but maintain a Judeo-Christian orientation. Many go through periodic religious crisis in their own lives (just as you and I) and keep their practice of therapy separate from their religious life. In a recent study by the American Psychiatric Association, only one out of every four psychiatrists listed himself as "atheistic," one third list themselves as "agnostic," and two-fifths list themselves as "theistic." Forty percent of psychiatrists attend church regularly or occasionally. Fifty-three percent send their children to religious schools. Twelve percent of the psychiatrists surveyed provided some type of service to religious groups. Some, however, do accept a particular form of psychotherapy with "religious zeal." These practitioners are to be feared both by the Christian community and the psychotherapeutic community. They do little to advance our knowledge of human behavior and fail to help their patients because of their stagnant orientations. For example, some have made psychoanalysis not only a therapeutic technique but a philosophy of life. God has been replaced by Freud as the ultimate authority and his writings become "the word." This type of psychotherapeutic approach is not only anti-Christian but antiscientific as well. Fortunately such individuals make up a minority of practicing psychotherapists. Unfortunately, the public often forms its image of psychiatry and clinical psychology from their practices. For example, most people envision every psychiatrist with a couch. Only a few ever use a couch in therapy and most of us have never owned one!

A competent therapist or counselor will call upon the religious life of his client as a source of strength. There may be problems that an individual is experiencing in his religious life that the therapist will find useful to explore and discuss, but these discussions should never challenge the basic tenets of one's faith.

An Ethical Therapist

Physicians, upon receiving their medical degrees, repeat the Oath of Hippocrates. Parts of this oath are especially pertinent in selecting a therapist. "I will follow that method of treatment which, according to my ability and judgment, I consider for the benefit of my patients and abstain from whatever is deleterious and mischievous . . . With purity and holiness I will pass my life and practice my art . . . Whatever, in connection with my professional practice, or not in connection with it, I may see or hear in the lives of men which ought not to be spoken abroad I will not divulge." The ingredients of the ethical therapist were never better spoken. They include competence, honesty, morality, confidentiality, and always putting the best interests of the patient first. The consumers of the mental health profession's services should expect nothing less. But Hippocrates was not the only one to enumerate the qualities of a servant of man. Paul, in 1 Timothy 3:1–13, in listing the qualities of the bishop (elder) and deacon in the church, reminded us of the characteristics of an ethical leader.

An Adequately Trained Therapist

Many different professionals and nonprofessionals are engaged in the practice of counseling and psychotherapy. Each profession has its own credentials for competence to practice therapy within that profession. Though orientations vary greatly between professions and appreciably within professions, each has rather strict guidelines for anyone wishing to "hang out his shingle." Let us look at a number of these professions and their requirements for certification of competence.

Psychiatry. Every psychiatrist has attended medical school and has received an M.D. degree. In addition, he must complete four years of training in psychiatry following graduation from medical school. This training must take place in an approved "psychiatric residency." Though most residency programs are associated with a medical school (such as the Department of Psychiatry of Duke University School of Medicine), many excellent residencies are found in private and state mental hospitals or community mental health centers. Upon completion of this required training, a psychiatrist is considered "board eligible" and can begin practice with the sanction of the specialty of psychiatry. Most psychiatrists take "psychiatry boards" two years following the completion of their residency training and, if they pass, become diplomates of the American Board of Psychiatry and Neurology. One can become a member of the American Psychiatric Association, the largest and most influential organization of psychiatrists, while in residency training, but must complete his training in order to retain that membership. There are many smaller psychiatric organizations (The American Psychosomatic Society, the Southern Psychiatric Association) that have similar, but often more stringent, requirements for membership.

It must be remembered that the only license in the medical profession is that granted for the practice of medicine in a given state. These licenses are obtainable in almost every state upon completing one year training after medical school. Therefore a physician can legally practice any specialty after this abbreviated training. One must be cautious of those who call themselves psychiatrists. I, therefore, would look further to see if the psychiatrist is board eligible (has completed four years of postgraduate training), board certified, and a member in good standing of local and/or national medical societies and associations. It may also be helpful to find if he has admitting privileges at a nearby hospital. Board eligibility is the most critical factor. Trainees in psychiatry (residents in a training program) may be available for psychotherapy at a lesser fee.

Clinical Psychology. A psychologist undergoes a different type of training. After completing the B.A. or B.S. degree, he must complete a master's degree and most obtain a Ph.D. or Ed.D. In order to be licensed to practice psychotherapy (or behavior therapy) in many states, he must undergo two additional years of training (including a psychology internship). With a master's degree, a psychologist can be licensed as a psychological examiner (which involves the administration and evaluation of psychological tests), but this does not allow him to practice psychotherapy. Upon completion of postdoctoral training, the clinical psychologist undergoes a written examination in the state where he chooses to practice.

The largest professional group of psychologists is the American Psychological Association, but this organization, for the most part, consists of psychologists who are not in practice. Instead, they are engaged in research and/or teaching.

Many so-called psychologists are engaged in therapies such as Transactional Analysis (TA) or Gestalt Therapy. The mainstream of psychology is concerned about those who practice such therapy because of the less rigorous training and certification required of practitioners. For example, some practitioners may feel themselves capable of setting up a practice, of say TA, after attending a two-week workshop with no formal educational background. These individuals may be well-meaning but suffer from the same problems as any untrained therapist. It should be said that the practitioners of TA are recognizing the problem of poorly-trained therapists and are making efforts to institutionalize the specialty. However, their efforts are quite weak compared to the mainstream of clinical psychology.

The most important qualifications to consider in a clinical psychologist are an academic degree (usually a Ph.D.) and a state license.

Social Work. The social worker, upon completing a B.A. or a B.S. degree, must have a M.S.W. or D.S.W.

degree to practice therapy. The M.S.W. degree is usually a two-year program with significant clinical experience under supervision. Upon completion of their
degrees, many social workers continue to obtain clinical supervision for an additional two years, undergo
an exam, and then are certified by the Academy of
Certified Social Workers (A.C.S.W.). In addition they
belong to the National Association of Social Workers
(N.A.S.W.).

Many individuals are hired by state, county, and
city departments of social service as social workers
and are assigned a case load of individuals who receive
continuing public services (welfare payments). It is
the social workers' duty to maintain contact with
these individuals and help them with the problems
of living that they may face. Most of the social workers
have a B.A. or B.S. degree only and are not involved
in the practice of psychotherapy. They are not trained
as therapists and must be distinguished from individuals who possess an M.S.W. degree. They are more
properly called case workers.

Social workers may set up a practice of marital
and family therapy. Yet there is no generally recognized formal licensing or certification for the specific
practice of marital and family therapy. Indeed, members of many specialties practice this type of therapy.
There is a nationwide Organization of Marriage and
Family Counselors which has a multidisciplinary
membership.

In considering the qualifications of a social

worker, the possession of an M.S.W. degree and membership in the N.A.S.W. would be the most critical factors.

Pastoral Counseling. Pastoral counseling as a specialty has become much more institutionalized over the past few years. Schools of pastoral counseling have developed throughout the country. Many ministers, weighted under by counseling problems, are returning to these schools for further training. Though the orientation of these schools may vary greatly, the general curriculum consists of course work in counseling theory, field placement (such as in a hospital), and supervision. There is an American Association of Pastoral Counselors that sets rather rigorous requirements for certification. These requirements include a college undergraduate degree, a seminary theological degree, three years as a recognized minister, priest, or rabbi and many hours of supervision in counseling. The training of a pastoral counselor involves little emphasis on the religious issues involved in counseling and is similar in many ways to the training of the psychologist or social worker. The religious orientation of a pastoral counselor may range from fundamentalistic to agnostic.

Needless to say, many ministers engaged in counseling have not undergone the training described above. Different models of training have developed in the more conservative theological schools (such as Fuller Theological Seminary, Trinity Theological Seminary in Chicago, and Abilene Christian University). These schools have developed both undergraduate and graduate courses in counseling. In addition, they have placed great emphasis on special workshops and training sessions. The graduate degrees offered are varied (B.D., M.A.) and usually represent a range of theological studies. Specialization is possible, and one can major in psychotherapy. New national organizations are growing out of this conservative tradition of Christian counseling, such as the Christian Association for Psychological Studies. Journals concerned with the dissemination of information on Christian psychology from a more conservative viewpoint are beginning to appear (*The Journal of Psychology and Theology*). As can be seen, fundamentalistic and evangelical religious groups have become progressively more interested in psychology, psychotherapy, and counseling. We may expect standards for certification of competence to appear in the near future, but never to the extent seen in the professions mentioned previously.

Lay Counseling. A new (but in fact very old) concept of counseling is beginning to develop in the more conservative and evangelical denominations. Christians are, once again, taking James seriously when he said, "Confess your sins to one another, and pray for one another, that you may be healed" (Jas. 5:16). Naturally, Christians have been counseling one another through the centuries. Many Christians have an innate ability and, with experience, are able to render a definite service to their cohorts. What is new is that some are seeking brief training experiences. For example, many Christian communities have established telephone counseling ministries. Following the pattern of the nationwide organization, Contact Teleministry, Christians from all walks of life enter training sessions in counseling. These sessions usually last for two hours once a week and extend through one semester. The curriculum includes lectures on mental illness, grief, and sexual problems, coupled with practiced-oriented workshops in telephone counseling. Once the course is completed, the individuals volunteer their time to man the phones of the counseling center. An important offshoot of such experiences is that these individuals become remarkably proficient in their ability to handle crisis situations. This, in turn, allows them to become valuable counseling resources in their individual congregations. Other models have been developed whereby lay members of a congregation obtain useful counseling skills and, in turn, are used, informally, as confidants and counselors to their fellow Christians.

Such individuals rarely request a fee and the formal rules of the counseling and therapeutic relationship (as described below) do not apply. Lay counselors are subject to the same inadequacies as any counselor with little training and should, above all, recognize their limitations. Yet we must not forget the biblical precedent and practical importance of these persons within the church.

This list does not exhaust the types of professionals and nonprofessionals involved in counseling and psychotherapy (nor the types of certification and requirements for certification). Yet, I hope this will serve as a guide to the Christian who seeks the services of a qualified therapist. These are the types of credentials that the wise consumer should consider.

Negotiate a Treatment Contract

Physicians commonly call those individuals who receive care or treatment a patient (a person who receives action or is affected). We are coming upon an age, however, in which the individual receiving care is not a passive recipient of the care of the physician but an active participant in a joint therapeutic process. An example of such active participation is the patient with diabetes. He regulates his diet, checks his urine for sugar, and self-medicates himself with insulin. Such active participation on the part of the patient is nowhere better seen than in the psychosocial therapies. In fact, the social workers have adopted the word *client* (or customer) to describe the recipients of their services.

Psychiatric treatment is like any other business transaction. A relationship is formed between two mutually consenting parties to a defined end. The therapist should agree to:

1. Be available at a certain time each week to the client (and to the client alone unless group or family therapy is the mode of treatment).

2. Use his professional abilities to help the client to understand a given problem and/or to learn new behaviors.

3. Advise the client of the possible outcomes of a given treatment modality.

4. Advise the client at any point in the therapeutic process when further treatment is to no avail.

5. Refer the client to other resources if such resources would be valuable to the client in addition to or instead of the prescribed treatment.

6. Perform all services in an ethical manner.

The client who wishes to receive services agrees to: (1) Pay the therapist a predetermined fee for service. (2) Cooperate in the therapeutic process.

The following example illustrates the process of developing a treatment contract. A middle-aged woman goes to a psychiatrist because she has been very depressed over the past three months. She has lost weight, has difficulty sleeping, and has developed a poor self-concept. Her husband has been less attentive to her recently, and she feels his inattention may be contributing to her depressed feelings. The psychiatrist agrees that she has correctly sought help for her problem. After a period of evaluation (usually one to three sessions), the psychiatrist tells her the following.

"You are suffering from a depressive reaction. Though it is not critical, it appears serious enough to warrant treatment. Because this depression is partly based on a physiologic reaction within your body, you would benefit from a medication. I will give you a prescription for a drug, called an antidepressant, that should help you. The drug will take about three weeks to take effect and the chances are very much in your favor that this medication will help you. You should expect to have improved sleep and appetite, and more energy and the depressed feeling will lift gradually. Once the depression has improved, it will be important for you to continue taking this medication for an additional six months to prevent a recurrence of the depression.

"However, from what you tell me, the relationship between you and your husband is not good, and I believe this is also having an effect upon your feelings. Because of the nature of the problem, I believe you could benefit from a course of brief psychotherapy. I would like to suggest meeting once a week for forty-five minutes for eight consecutive weeks. During this time I will monitor your response to the antidepressant medication. In addition, I could help you to better understand your relationship with your husband. I suspect that some of the problems you have had in this relationship are associated with difficulties that you have experienced in the past. By talking about your present and past experiences, I can help you to explore new ways to interact with your husband. I do not promise that you will never become depressed again. However, I believe the chances are excellent that you will recover from your present depressive episode and that the period of psychotherapy will help you to prevent such episodes in the future.

"My fee is thirty-five dollars per session. It will be payable at the end of each month. I could arrange to see you at this same time each week over the next eight weeks."

That is a reasonable statement of what a psychiatrist can offer this client as the most appropriate therapy for her condition. As you can see, it is a combined treatment approach (drug therapy and psychotherapy) that is self-limiting. He does not promise her a total cure. Total cures are rarities in emotional illness. Neither does he require that she continue to see him indefinitely. The prognosis in overcoming a circumscribed depressive episode in the middle years is quite good. Therefore the psychiatrist can afford to be optimistic and self-limiting in his approach. More chronic problems may involve a contract requiring continual care from a psychiatrist (treating someone with chronic schizophrenia). Other treatment contracts may involve frequent sessions over a long period of time (four sessions a week for three to four years in psychoanalysis). These are not unlike the frequent and continued medical attention required for patients with kidney failure, who must undergo hemodialysis three times a week for the remainder of their lives.

Once the therapist has offered his evaluation of what treatment modalities would be most appropriate and his own willingness to render such therapies, the client has the right to accept or reject his offer. In the above example, the woman may agree totally with the psychiatrist. On the other hand, she may wish to explore whether she might benefit from the psychotherapy without the antidepressant medication. Regardless, a period of negotiations often takes place and a mutual agreement is fixed. Then the treatment process can proceed.

Unfortunately both clients and therapists often neglect establishing a treatment contract in the initial therapeutic sessions. It has been my experience that therapy often fails when no contract has been established. The reasons for this are numerous. For example, avoiding a treatment contract breeds lack of responsibility on the part of both client and therapist. The therapist may have unrealistic expectations as to what he can expect from the client (that she will continue to come to the sessions indefinitely). In turn, the client may have unrealistic expectations as to what she can expect from the therapist (that he will spend extra time with her or that he will not charge her for the sessions). When these mutual expectations are not forthcoming, both parties become discouraged and the therapy is greatly hindered.

A treatment contract breeds responsibility on the part of both therapist and client. This adult interaction, in itself, is often quite therapeutic for the individual who has emotional difficulties related to immature behavior.

Establish a Fee

"For the scripture says, 'You shall not muzzle an ox when it is treading out the grain,' and, 'The laborer deserves his wages' " (1 Tim. 5:18). Counseling is work! The practice of psychotherapy can be very rewarding, but it is not fun. As with any profession, the practitioner should receive a just compensation for his efforts.

The fees for counseling may vary greatly. This variation does not necessarily represent the competency of the therapist but is more likely a representation of the training of the therapist and the type of therapy he practices. For example, a psychiatrist who holds a M.D. degree and has at least eight years of training after undergraduate school will usually charge more than a psychologist or social worker with fewer years of training. This, however, is not always the case. A psychologist who specializes in a popular type of therapy and is well known for his work may command a higher fee. Since there are generally no established levels of fees, the law of supply and demand often influences the fee scale in a given area. Fees in clinics such as a community mental health center or the psychiatric outpatient department of a major hospital tend to be much lower, but such clinics may have long waiting lists or limited forms of therapy.

Fees for psychotherapy are generally open to negotiation and many practitioners have a sliding scale (a percentage of the maximum fee based on an individual's income). Fees may also vary with different geographic locations. Private practitioners in Boston will command a higher fee than practitioners in a rural Southern community. Many practitioners will carry a certain number of clients at reduced rates, regardless of the fee scale of that area.

Though major medical insurance covers the cost of most inpatient psychiatric hospital expenses, few insurance policies cover outpatient counseling and then only from psychiatrists. Therefore, unlike most medical expenses, the cost of psychotherapy must come out of the pocket of the client. It is for this reason that psychotherapy fees are subject to negotiation, unlike most medical treatments. Regardless, the final fee is that which is agreed upon by the therapist and clients.

"Why pay a fee at all?" "Can't I find someone to counsel me for free?" "Isn't paying for a therapist just a waste of money?" Once it has been determined that some type of mental health service is needed, I strongly recommend that a client pay *something*. The reasons are two-fold. First, in the mental health profession, you generally get what you pay for (free advice is worth about what it costs). The second reason, though, may be even more important. Psychotherapy, unlike most services rendered, requires the cooperation and, often, the active participation of the client in order to be effective. The client, as well as the therapist, must *work* toward a common goal. This work requires motivation. One way to ensure motivation is to make an investment. An investment of money, as well as time, is often the key to success. I have accepted young adults as clients in the past and have required them to pay the fee themselves rather than borrow the money from their parents. Though I had to reduce my fee in such cases, I was much more satisfied with the results of the therapy.

To paraphrase a sign at the cashier's office in the Metropolitan Museum of Art in New York City, if you wish to ensure a successful psychotherapy, you may pay whatever fee you and your therapist agree upon, but you must pay something.

Seek Spiritual Support

The Christian will most often find that his emotional problems are associated with spiritual problems. Such an individual may wish to talk with a minister or church leader. Spiritual support and counsel must be coordinated with psychotherapy. The therapist and minister should be in contact with one another. If not, at least they should each be aware of the other's activities in the care of the client. If conflicts in the counsel of the spiritual adviser and the psychotherapist arise, it is *imperative* that they meet together. Usually these differences can be worked out easily once the parties involved meet face to face but rarely can they be worked out when messages are being carried back and forth by the client. If they do not meet, the psychotherapy often becomes ineffective.

Unfortunately, there is a definite resistance on the part of both religious and mental health workers to meet together. I believe this is inexcusable. Neither the church nor the mental health profession can afford to work in a vacuum. Each is concerned with the care of the whole person. The overlap of emotional and spiritual problems is significant. Competency impels cooperation and mutual understanding.

Know When to Stop

Counseling, and psychotropic medications for that matter, are like any other forms of treatment. Sometimes they just do not work. Our Lord has given us the intelligence to determine whether a treatment experience is effective or not. Once you have given psychotherapy your best effort (which may take months) and no results are forthcoming, know when to stop.

One of the most difficult aspects of psychotherapy is termination. In other words, how do you stop the process once it has begun? Most often the client stops coming to the sessions or leaves a message that he is quitting. Both the therapist and the client feel badly about their work together and therefore feel badly about each other. These bad feelings can be alleviated if the client and therapist can openly talk about "calling it quits." Talking about the unpleasant is never easy, but the client will feel better afterwards. Possibly the therapist is thinking the same thing and will be relieved if he learns that the client is not angry with him but has made a realistic appraisal of their joint efforts. That appraisal leads to the conclusion that further treatment if not useful. Such actions on the part of the client and therapist allow them to part friends. The anger initially directed toward the therapist is replaced by the much more tolerable emotion of disappointment that the efforts were ineffective.

The reasons that therapy does not work in a given situation are numerous. Possibly the client had unreasonable expectations about what could be accomplished by therapy, or a change in therapeutic approach may be needed. Occasionally personality conflicts arise between the client and therapist that cannot be resolved. Rarely does religious conflicts interfere with the progress of therapy. But for many problems there may be (and often is) a point where acceptance is the answer. As Paul said, "I have learned, in whatever state I am, to be content" (Phil. 4:11). Therapy may then have been valuable in helping one come to a point of acceptance.

4

THE ROLE OF THE SPIRITUAL COMMUNITY

The local spiritual community can undertake and practice many activities that will greatly facilitate the healing resources available to troubled Christians. The church, as an institution, must become involved in the ministry to the emotionally disturbed. God developed a *plan* (a strategy, if you will) by which all men might be saved (his goal). "This Jesus, delivered up according to the definite plan and foreknowledge of God" (Acts 2:23). If one sets a goal, such as developing an effective counseling ministry in the church, one would be well-advised to develop a strategy for implementing this goal. Though much counseling in the church takes place in an informal atmosphere, support systems for counseling can be enhanced greatly by proper planning. What are the ingredients of a strategy for developing an effective Christian counseling ministry?

Identify Capable Mental Health Workers

If a Christian who requires professional help comes to a minister or church leader, that leader should be able to refer the troubled Christian to a

capable professional (Christian or non-Christian de-
pending upon available resources). These requests,
because they are so frequent, should never come as
a surprise.

Church leaders can survey the mental health facilities in their area. Public clinics and hospitals, such
as a community mental health center, a child guidance
clinic, or the psychiatric ward of a local hospital, will
often provide written materials describing their services. In addition, they often arrange time to acquaint
a representative of a congregation or religious organization with their program. We should take advantage
of these opportunities for touring facilities and meeting with mental health workers. Questions can be
asked about referral procedures, therapeutic orientations, and coordination with other service agencies.
I have found that most clinics and institutions are
quite happy to meet with designated representatives
of community organizations such as churches, with
time being the only limiting factor. These facilities
and programs have a need to build good, solid public
relations with the community.

Gathering information about private practitioners is a more difficult task. The first step would be
for all the religious leaders in a given area to share
their experiences in working with the private sector.
Usually a group of names emerge that many have
found to be competent and financially reasonable. The
range of professionals that emerge from such a pool-
ing of information may be quite varied. One Christian

community may identify a number of psychiatrists but no marital counselors. Another group of church leaders may not identify a competent psychiatrist, but a series of social workers and clinical psychologists that are acceptable. Lists of professionals can be assembled and good or bad experiences can be exchanged on an ongoing basis. Naturally, no one professional is uniformly successful, and every professional will receive "bad press." General trends, however, can be identified over time.

If a church leader has a number of marital problems that he would like to refer for counseling, he may contact a professional in the area about the feasibility of referral. It is not beyond reason that he might arrange a meeting to discuss referral procedures and to learn more of the counselor's therapeutic orientation. Unless the counselor has a full practice, he most likely will jump at the advantage of becoming acquainted with a potential referral source. In the final analysis, however, the Christian community must take the initiative in identifying competent and acceptable professionals to serve the emotional needs of its members.

Establish Relationships with Mental Health Workers

Paul said, "I have become all things to all men" (1 Cor. 9:22). In order to be effective as an evangelist, he saw a need to be adaptable. This adaptability allowed him to make contact with those "under the

law" and "outside the law" (v. 20). In turn, these con-
tacts allowed him to lead these groups to Christ. Yet
he was capable of being adaptable because "I am free
from all men" (1 Cor. 9:19). The Christian does not
need to be afraid of the mental health worker, yet I
see many fellow church members who appear awed
by psychiatry and psychology. The fear of the field
is often translated into a separatist and aloof attitude.
Regardless of what ostensible reason is given for this
separatist attitude, the implied message is, "If I, as
a Christian, associate with and work with a psychiatrist, I will lose my own identity." Nothing could
be further from the truth. We are *free*. We have an
identity and role of which we can be proud. The
Christian community always has an important role
to play in the total care of the emotionally-disturbed
Christian. We have something to contribute to the
emotionally disturbed that will be recognized by others as being of value. These valuable resources include
a supportive community, manpower, finances, and
auxiliary services such as financial advisers, educational advisers, wise and sensitive individuals in leadership positions. Therefore, we as a Christian community, can face the mental health community with
boldness.

      Yet we are not the only ones afraid. Many mem-
bers of the mental health community are equally
afraid of the Christian community. We must help
them to overcome their fears of working with Christians. What are these fears? The general concerns of

the mental health community are that Christians are inflexible, that they are only trying to convert people, that they only wish to make people feel more guilt, that they cannot work with others, and, most of all, that they wish to deny the good works of the behavioral sciences and wish to destroy the profession. Can these fears be alleviated?

The Cole Mill Road Church of Christ in Durham, North Carolina, initiated an experiment two years ago. The hypothesis was simple but unique: A church, a community mental health center, civic groups, and the state government can work together to provide a much desired service in Durham County. The community desperately needed a group home for emotionally-disturbed adolescent girls. Getting representatives from each of these groups to sit down together in the same room was quite an accomplishment. The greater accomplishment, however, was establishment of the home itself. At present, the home is operating smoothly and effectively. The church has been allowed to carry on any programs in evangelistic instruction it wishes, within reason. Girls in the home attend church, and the other agencies involved with the program are most happy that religious instructions have become an integral part of the program. Naturally the home continues to have periodic problems, but the fact that it is functioning today is a testimony that Christians and the mental health profession *can* work together effectively. Initial fears on both sides have been, for the most part, extinguished, yet neither group has lost its identity or primary purpose.

It is not necessary for every Christian community to erect such an elaborate working relationship as the one just described. Each church can, however, establish a working relationship with mental health workers that have been identified as useful to the community. How does one go about establishing such relationships?

1. If you, as a minister or church leader, have been counseling with an emotionally disturbed church member who is seeing a secular counselor or psychotherapist, you may feel free to contact the therapist and inform him of your relationship with this client. Let the therapist know that you are most concerned with the welfare of the client and do not wish to work at crosscurrents with the therapist.

2. If you have the permission of the church member, you may volunteer information and impressions that you have gained during your relationship with the church member.

3. You may ask the therapist (again with the permission of the church member) if there is anything that you might do to facilitate the healing of the emotional problems.

4. If a conflict appears to be arising, you might suggest that you and the therapist meet for a conference to discuss the impending difficulties.

As the above relationship develops, the minister or church leader should never indicate that he plans to cease contact with the church member or "step out of the picture." Yet there may be certain subjects that, after discussion with the therapist, are referred back to the therapist. For example, a minister and therapist may agree that a particular sexual problem will be discussed only during psychotherapy. If the church member brings the subject up with the church leader, the leader may then say, "We [the church leader, the therapist, *and* the church member] have agreed that you will discuss that subject only with your therapist. There are many other things that we may talk about." On the other hand, it may be mutually agreed that certain religious issues will be discussed only with the church leader. Such a division of labor does not divide the client but does diminish the possibilities of role confusion and the playing of one counselor against another. If the client is a particularly manipulative individual, such communication and division of labor may be vital to the success of the total healing of the disturbed individual.

Such relationships do not evolve easily between groups that have a history of being at war with one another. They literally have to be hammered out over time. Yet their potential for service to the emotionally-disturbed Christian make the effort infinitely worthwhile.

Develop an Atmosphere of Support

An effective Christian community is a supportive community. What are the ingredients of such a community? How can we, as individual Christians, contribute to an atmosphere of support?

Establish a True Fellowship

What constitutes a fellowship? We belong to many different groups in our day-to-day activities (families, professions, community, political parties). A true fellowship, however, is much more than an arbitrary assignment of categories. The group members must meet together (Heb. 10:25), be open with one another (Jas. 5:16), forgive one another (Col. 3:13), and be honest with one another (Eph. 4:25–26). Only when the members of the Christian community practice these activities can an atmosphere of fellowship develop.

Establish a Giving and Receiving Environment

In this fiercely independent society we live in, learning to give and receive is one of our most difficult tasks. Ironically, most of us have more trouble receiving than giving. Our pride will often prevent us from asking for the help we need. Then we wonder why others don't call on us for help. I, personally, am much more likely to ask for the assistance of those who will allow me to return the favor. There is not one of us who cannot use the assistance of fellow Christians. We may ask for help in moving a piano, assistance in filing a tax return, or prayers for healing. Once we have set the precedent of asking for help, people are more likely to turn to us in a time of need.

The professional psychotherapist does not ask for counsel from his client for very special reasons. Formal therapy is therefore unique, a sort of one-way street. Christian interaction, however, *must* operate on a very different premise. It must be a *sharing* community rather than a community divided into counselors and counselees. We "confess your sins to one another" (Jas. 5:16) and "bear one another's burdens" (Gal. 6:2). Giving and receiving are hallmarks of the truly supportive Christian community.

We must also be ready to help those with even the most mundane requests. An emotionally-disturbed individual may be literally crying for someone to talk with but, at the same time, be suspicious of the intent of those around. He may then test a fellow Christian with a superficial request ("Will you help me move my couch?" "Will you give me a lift home?"). Many Christians view such requests as being beneath their dignity, yet would jump at the opportunity to counsel a brother in need. But they never pass the first test of a good counselor, willingness to help. If we are willing to help move that couch or to drive that person home, we often find the troubled person opening up to us the suffering he is experiencing.

Use Available Resources Effectively. Every congregation of Christians has members with various talents and abilities. We must remember that emotional illness may be caused by any number of etiological agents. True stress from the environment may be a significant causative agent. This stress may be in the form of poverty, legal problems, a need for household repairs, or a need for recreation. We can use our law-

yers, doctors, accountants, and/or repairmen, to meet
these very specific problems.

Use the Pulpit to Encourage Sharing. The demeanor
of the minister in the pulpit often "sets the tone"
of a given congregation of Christians. A minister can
demonstrate his care for his flock, or he can vent his
frustration at their negligence. He can speak of "your"
problems or he can speak of "our" problems. He can
discuss abstract theological doctrines or he can discuss
the very real day-to-day problems that every Christian
faces. He can realistically accept the many emotional
problems that exist within his congregation or he can
downplay such problems as "unchristian." He can
preach despair or he can preach hope. The minister's
attitude toward emotional problems, the emotionally
disturbed, and the mental health profession will be
translated into sermons week after week.

In the "best of all possible worlds" (as Candide
would say), a minister should not have such a profound influence over a congregation. We must face
the fact that this is *not* the best of all worlds and
that the message from the pulpit each Sunday morning is by far the most important policy statement of
a given religious group and will almost always reflect
the attitudes and actions of that group. To develop
a true atmosphere of support, we must reach the men
in the pulpit with our message.

There are certainly other activities that would
enhance a fellowship conducive to effective Christian
healing of emotional disturbances. The above, how-

ever, should provide a starting point for each Christian community to reconsider the supportive aspects of that community.

Establish a Prayer Ministry

"Of course we will pray for you." Prayer would appear to be the easiest and most natural endeavor to help the emotionally disturbed. Yet we often get lulled into a lazy and ineffective prayer life. The church, in general, has let a once-excellent idea, the prayer meeting, degenerate into just another period of fellowship and preaching. We, as individual Christians, rarely get down on our knees but choose to pray in our minds as we go to sleep. Such prayers quickly slip into daydreaming and rarely are brought to conclusion. Grace at meals often becomes a formality with little or no originality or thought, as evidenced by the fact that we occasionally cannot remember if we have said grace or not. We believe in prayer, but prayer takes *work*. Many of us do not choose to make the effort to seriously develop our prayer life. If a congregation desires to establish a prayer ministry, it must count the cost of such an effort. Some ingredients of a successful endeavor in prayer for the emotionally disturbed are discussed below.

Pray with the Individual Requesting or Needing Our Prayers. When someone comes to us and asks us to pray for them, we often say, "Of course I will" and never give it another thought. We do not take such requests seriously, and the disturbed do not request our prayers seriously. They may have no intention of changing their lives and actually have no true belief in the power of prayer, but ask because asking for prayers is a right thing to do at church. A more serious response to a request for prayer might be, "I will certainly pray for you, but I want those prayers to be effective. Will you tell me what I should pray for? Will you pray with me?" Such statements accomplish two things. First, the Christian making such statements accepts the responsibility of taking some time and making some effort to effect a change. Second, the one requesting prayers is forced to take some responsibility in making such a request. At this point "the ante is upped" in that a casual remark has become a serious mutual endeavor.

The advantages of praying for an individual with that individual physically present are many. If such a person can humble himself to listen to prayers for himself by others, he has taken a great step forward. In addition, he is supported in his difficulties by others and does not have to face the challenges of life alone. Prayers by a group (provided the group is not too large) will unite a group behind a particular goal, such as the healing and support of a fellow group member. The ultimate advantage, however, of praying with someone else is the facilitation of communication. Prayer is one of the most intimate activities in which two or more individuals can be engaged. The disordered communication of the emotionally disturbed can be replaced by the honest and sincere communication necessary in praying together. God will certainly hear such prayers.

Praying with someone, however, implies more than just being physically with them during prayer. Effective prayers are coordinated prayers. We cannot always assume that we are praying for the same thing our brother is praying for. Mary may come and ask you to pray for her separated husband, John. You may pray that John returns home to Mary. Mary may be praying that John "really gets what's coming to him." Praying for John can mean different things to different people. The only way I know to coordinate our prayers is to talk about the particular needs for which an individual is requesting our prayers.

Pray at a Definite Time. Praying successfully is a skill. The only way one can master a skill is to practice it regularly not on a hit-or-miss basis. If prayer is to become a consistent part of our lives, we must condition ourselves to pray at certain times of the day. Many select the time just before going to sleep or the time just after they arise in the mornings to pray. For others there are more effective times for prayer (that fifteen quiet minutes at the office before your secretary gets to work or the time right after the kids have left for school). The time for prayer will be different for each individual. Establishing a regular time is the most important factor.

A big step toward developing a prayer ministry is setting aside a time when groups of Christians can meet together to pray. Like any task force, such a group must sacrifice time and energy to achieve a certain goal. I suspect that if such a group is to survive, it will need to keep abreast of the success of its prayers. Some groups have even gone so far as to keep a notebook listing the date the prayer for an individual was initially offered and the date the prayer was answered. The results of prayer are visible and any prayer group should periodically review previous prayers and thank God for the prayers he has answered.

Pray for Specific Needs. So often we "pray for Mary, John, Bill, and Alice," but never state what we are praying for. God wishes to be our confidant. He wants us to feel free to open up the inner thoughts and feelings that trouble us. Yet we often pray to God as if he were a casual acquaintance, speaking in generalities and formalities. We don't get down to business with our prayers about ourselves or others. Once we become more specific, God can (1) help us to understand what possible choices are available in a given situation and (2) answer a definite request.

The individual who prays a specific prayer must seriously consider the object of his prayer. An old saying that is particularly popular in psychiatric circles is, "You had better be careful what you pray for because your prayers might be answered." Certain men and women literally pray for years that they get into medical school. They never give serious thought to what it means to be a doctor and never take the time to find out about a life in medicine. Their prayers are answered upon entering medical school, but they are miserable in the anatomy and biochemistry labs. They are even more miserable on the medical wards and would give anything to be somewhere else. They prayed with Spirit but not with understanding.

The emotionally disturbed often request something without giving serious thought to the implications of their request. Plunging headlong into a particular course of action, they refuse to listen to alternatives. Their prayers may be answered, but they are more miserable at the end than when they began.

Pray with a Positive Attitude. "And whatever you ask in prayer, you will receive, if you have faith." (Matt. 21:22). Faith in God and faith in ourselves through the Spirit of God are necessary ingredients of a successful prayer ministry. The church should not only pray for the emotionally disturbed but it should pray for an effective healing environment to exist within its fellowship also. Many of us have little faith in our potential as a congregation to accomplish the will of God. The fractured relationships, cliques, and personal quarrels discourage us to the point of despair. We must never forget that God can succeed where man will fail in effecting a healing fellowship.

Pray with an Attitude of Surrender. "Nevertheless, not as I will, but as thou wilt" (Matt. 26:39). When we pray to God about a particular matter, we must literally turn that matter over to God. This requires a significant degree of flexibility, a willingness to listen to others, a true desire to change, and trust in a being other than ourselves. Each of these qualities is an important plus in successful therapy of the emotionally disturbed. With such qualities intact within the personality, few disturbances can be permanently damaging to the whole person.

The Christian community must also be willing to pray with an attitude of surrender. To effect a healing ministry, plans may have to change, leadership roles may have to be altered, and occasionally great sacrifices must be made. The community may be called upon to contribute a considerable amount of money to support a brother in an institution if this is the only successful therapy available for that individual. Many counseling hours at odd times of the day may be required in another case. In yet another, members of the church may have to demonstrate infinite patience in working with a very dependent and clinging fellow member. Emotional problems that are years in the making do not correct themselves overnight. We must surrender our fantasized beliefs in instant cures of some problems and accept the slow but sure healing that God provides.

Prayer can change lives! Prayer can heal! Yet no tool so powerful can be easily mastered. We must *work* to develop a successful prayer ministry in the church.

Develop Effective Counselors Within the Christian Community

Each congregation or fellowship of Christians has counselors and counselees. Certain individuals, for various reasons, are gifted in listening to the problems of the emotionally disturbed and are noted for their wise and appropriate counsel. These counselors may be church leaders, community leaders within the church, professional counselors who are active Christians (ranging from psychiatrists to personnel managers), or housewives and businessmen. God has provided such individuals with innate abilities to help the troubled of this world. Such Christians would never dream of "hanging out a shingle" but provide an essential function within the Christian fellowship. As a congregation of Christians considers how it may develop its counseling ministry, it does not have to start from scratch. Those in the fellowship who serve as counselors should be identified as valuable resources in whatever program is initiated. In fact, the preexisting network of counseling should be identified and strengthened as the backbone of any program.

How are such individuals identified? We can use the techniques of the systems analyst by asking certain key questions.

1. Who would I turn to if I had an emotional problem?
2. Who do I feel I could trust?
3. Who are the overt and covert leaders of the congregation? (Who do people usually turn to for advice?)
4. Do those in trouble turn for help inside or outside the congregation?

If a congregation is honestly willing to ask such questions, certain names will turn up again and again. These individuals are the unofficial counselors in the congregation and should be recognized as such.

The next step is for these individuals to meet together. We must remember that such a meeting is not a natural or easy endeavor for these counselors. Their own counseling ministry, however informal, is certainly a very personal matter to them. They may fear that information revealed to them in confidence by their troubled friends is in danger. At the same time, they may not wish to publicize their activities for fear of criticism. Many may feel there is nothing to be learned or gained by sharing with others their counseling activities. A slow, careful, and sensitive approach to these hesitations will usually facilitate more openness about individual counseling experiences. Most counselors have a feeling of loneliness in their activities, especially when they are faced with a particularly difficult and sensitive problem.

Whenever Christian counselors from the same fellowship meet together, confidentiality does become a key issue. Anyone who agrees to listen to someone else in confidence is obliged to do just that. Particular problems can be disguised enough in group meetings to maintain confidentiality and yet serve as the basis of a useful discussion. Groups soon learn to use such case presentations as focal points of discussion and quickly lose their curiosity about the particular individuals involved.

Meetings of counselors within a congregation should not be publicized and should be as informal as possible. If other members of the congregation become curious as to the purpose of these meetings, a simple statement usually suffices. "We are a group of Christians who are particularly interested in the problems of living and, in particular, how we might better minister to our fellow Christians. We have decided to meet regularly and to discuss these problems."

Such a group may undertake a more formal introduction into the theory and process of counseling. The elders and deacons of the Church of Christ in Durham, North Carolina, have considered undertaking a program of training in counseling principles and techniques. These theoretical considerations could then serve as a basis for discussing particular counseling problems (a discussion of the problem of alcoholism would be the nucleus for looking at individual experiences of counselors with alcoholic counselees). Such continuing education of church leaders may center around a particular book or a series of topics. Leadership in the discussion could be rotated. I believe that such discussions can be of definite benefit, even without the assistance of a trained professional. Errors and blind spots in counseling techniques are often brought to light during such discussions.

The most effective discussion groups are usually made up of six to eight individuals with a designated leader for each discussion. There should be a definite agenda, which may range from topic-oriented discussions to presenting a particularly thorny counseling problem on a rotating basis. The format should be informal, and an atmosphere of mutual support is essential. The attitude of each participant, including the leader, should be, "I will be a more effective counselor by sharing my successes and failures in counseling with my Christian friends. I will accept their confidences and will in turn trust their discretion."

An even more effective means of mutual support and another model that I have found to be highly effective is the area-wide, ongoing counseling seminar. Ministers, elders, and other counselors in churches from a given geographic area agree to meet together in groups of six to eight to discuss counseling problems. Many advantages are derived from having one representative of each congregation. It is less difficult to talk with someone outside the individual congregations about sensitive emotional issues within that congregation. Confidentiality becomes less of an issue. Opinions given are usually more objective and, therefore, more accurate. It is even possible for such groups to engage a professional consultant on a biweekly or monthly basis. Such a consultant's services could be paid for with a minimum expense by each seminar participant. Individual congregations could pick up the tab for their representative in the seminar (a small price to pay for a more effective counseling ministry). Such seminars are usually most effective when they are case centered. Individual participants can rotate each week in presenting a particular problem with which they have been working. New suggestions made during the seminar could be attempted in subsequent sessions with the disturbed counselee. The results of such interventions could be reported back to the seminar. This longitudinal view of emotional problems is invaluable in becoming an effective counselor. As seminar participants get to know and trust one another, the experience of sharing counseling experiences over time will become one of the most treasured and useful activities of the counselor.

A more serious and formal approach by the church is to develop and update undergraduate and graduate programs in Christian colleges and universities. Such programs should be supported and encouraged by the church, for only when a real need is expressed by the Christian community will our institutes of higher learning approach these problems seriously. Courses in counseling at many of our schools lack substance and clinical experience is virtually absent. Supervised counseling experience remains the most effective means of training. Such training usually requires cooperation with existing counseling centers and a graduate level of instruction. New and unusual approaches to training have been attempted by certain groups outside the university system. The Institutes of Religion and Health in New York City is a center of community psychiatry where individuals from varied backgrounds come together for one or two years of intensive training in counseling. The goal is to develop competent counselors who can render mental health services with a Christian orientation and at a cost not prohibitive to those who cannot afford private counseling.

Theoretical issues in Christianity and the behavioral sciences must be addressed by God-fearing and thoughtful individuals. New and comprehensive approaches to the body, mind, and spirit can stimulate each Christian to soberly consider his relationships with God, man, and self. There is much room for scholarly thought and writing in this critical area of the Christian experience.

The development of an annotated list of reading materials on counseling, therapy, and the theory of emotional illness is an additional step that a Christian community can take toward developing an effective counseling ministry. The book stores are replete with reading material on the problems of living. No one person can possible read all that is available. Unfortunately, most of what is available is not worth reading. If Christians could pool their knowledge and experiences in this area, valuable time could be saved, and the best resources could be identified and made available to those who counsel. Reading is a helpful way to increase one's ability as a counselor. Selective reading is even more helpful.

Many communities have education programs available in mental health that are of high quality and free. For example, the Center for Preventive Psychiatry in White Plains, New York, has published an excellent series of books for children on such childhood problems as handicaps, death and dying, and going to the hospital. They also present programs on various subjects to interested religious and civic groups free of charge. Though the information disseminated by such programs may not be entirely acceptable to the Christian viewpoint, I have usually found their input most helpful. Community programs about alcoholism and drug abuse are usually quite effective. The church should take advantage of such programs if it is to truly effect a counseling ministry.

In Conclusion

The church cannot ignore the emotional problems within its fellowship. They will not go away. I believe God would have us approach these problems with faith and reason. Accurate knowledge of mental illness and therapeutic forms coupled with effective planning can greatly facilitate the use of mental health resources in the community and the counseling resources within the church. Christians will never be required to compromise the centrality and supremacy of the basic message of the gospel (the salvation of the lost) to effect a counseling ministry. The counseling ministry is an adjunct to the church, a means to an end. An emotionally healthy community has much energy freed from dealing with internal conflict. This energy can be mobilized to press forward with our mission.

NOTES

1. S. H. Nelson and E. F. Torrey, "The Religious Functions of Psychiatry," *American Journal of Orthopsychiatry*, 43(3):362–367, 1973.

2. J. E. Adams, *Competent to Counsel* (Grand Rapids: Baker Book House, 1970).

3. Dorthea C. Leighton, *The Character of Danger: Psychiatric Symptoms in Selected Communities* (New York: Basic Books, 1963).

4. Eric Berne, *Games People Play* (New York: Grove Press, 1964).

5. Karl Menninger, *Whatever Became of Sin?* (New York: Hawthorne Books, Inc., 1973).

6. Alexander Campbell, *The Christian System in Reference to the Union of Christians and Restoration of Primitive Christianity, as Pled in the Current Reformation. History of Religion in America Series* (Nashville: Gospel Advocate Company, 1964).

7. Hal Lindsey and C. C. Carlson, *Satan Is Alive and Well on Planet Earth* (Grand Rapids: Zondervan, 1972).

8. E. F. Torrey, *The Mind Game: Witchdoctors and Psychiatry* (New York: Emerson Hall, 1972).

9. D. Blazer, "The Church and Modern Group Concepts," *Mission* 9:225, 1976.

10. J. B. Parker, D. G. Blazer, and L. Wyrick, "Anorexia Nervosa: A Combined Therapeutic Approach," *Southern Medical Association Journal* (in press).
11. Torrey, *The Mind Game*.

READING LIST

General

W. Glasser, *Mental Health or Mental Illness: Psychiatry for Practical Action* (New York: Harper and Row, 1961). A good introduction for any O. Q. Hyder, *The Christian Handbook of Psychiatry* (Old Tappan, New Jersey: Revell, 1971). An introduction to some of the more popular therapeutic modalities in psychiatry from the viewpoint of a Christian psychiatrist.

T. Lidz, *The Person: His Development Throughout the Life Cycle* (New York: Basic Books, 1968). The best introduction I know to the life cycle considering the viewpoints of Freud, Piaget, and Erikson along with other well-known theorists. The book reads very easily. Paul Tournier, *The Meaning of Persons* (New York: Harper and Row, 1957). A viewpoint of a well-known Christian psychiatrist on the makeup of the individual. This has been a very popular book in the past for Christian therapists.

Early Childhood

J. Dobson, *Dare to Discipline* (Wheaton, Illinois: Tyndale House, 1970). A very good approach to child rearing that emphasizes a consistent approach to discipline combined with love.

E. H. Erikson, *Childhood and Society* (New York: Norton, 1963). The most famous of Erikson's works, this book gives his view of the life cycle of the child. It is somewhat difficult to read but the insight gained by the counselor makes it worthwhile.

Selma H. Friaberg, *The Magic Years* (New York: Scribner's Sons, 1959). A good introduction to the thoughts and fantasies of the preschooler. H. G. Ginott, *Between Parent and Child* (New York: MacMillan, 1965). An excellent introduction to communication patterns between parents and children.

B. R. McCandless, *Childhood and Adolescence* (New York: Holt, Rinehart and Winston, 1961). A standard textbook on the normal development of the child considering both physical and psychological aspects. Benjamin Spock, *Baby and Child Care* (New York: Pocket Books, 1968). Regardless of his political views, this still remains a valuable resource on the normal development of a child. One does not have to follow his recommendations for punishment and discipline however.

Adolescence

Group for the Advancement of Psychiatry, *Normal Adolescence: Its Dynamics and Impact* (New York: Scribner's Sons, 1968). The best brief introduction to the physiologic and psychologic aspects of adolescence that I have read.

H. G. Ginott, *Between Parent and Teenager* (New York: MacMillan, 1969). More of Ginott's approach to communication.

I. Josselyn, *The Adolescent and His World* (New York: Family Service Association of America, 1952). A good introduction to the psychoanalytic views of adolescents with particular emphasis on such aspects of adolescence as hero worship and crushes.

Marriage and the Family

L. Christenson, *The Christian Family* (Minneapolis: Bethany Fellowship, 1971). A very popular book among Christians describing the commitment of the Christian family to the Lord.

R. Lofton Hudson, *Till Divorce Do Us Part* (Nashville: Thomas Nelson, 1974). A book worth reading. It deals with the meaning of divorce and the desirability of avoiding such marital terminations.

O. Q. Hyder, *The People You Live With* (Old Tappan, New Jersey: Revell, 1975). A superficial introduction to marital and family problems with Christians.

Judson T. Landis and Mary G. Landis, *Building a Successful Marriage*, Fourth Edition (Englewood Cliffs, New Jersey: Prentice-Hall, 1963). An old standard textbook on marriage and the family that continues to prove quite valuable.

David Mace and Vera Mace, *We Can Have Better Marriages* (Nashville: Abingdon, 1974). A book written by a couple known for their work in Christian marriages. This book points out the strengths of marriages.

Human Sexuality

F. Belliveau and L. Richcer, *Understanding Human Sexual Inadequacy* (Boston: Little, Brown and Company, 1970). A clear and simple explanation of the work of Masters and Johnson.

Eward Brecher and Ruth Brecher, *An Analysis of Human Sexual Response* (New York: The New American Library, 1966). Another excellent explanation of the work of Masters and Johnson.

S. A. Lewin and J. Gilmin, *Sex Without Fear* (New York: Medical Research Press, 1965). A good introduction for couples considering marriage.

R. L. Pettus, *As I See Sex Through the Bible* (Madison, Tennessee: Robert Pettus, 1973). This book, available on order from the author, is a very good and solid approach to human sexuality written by a member of the Church of Christ.

D. Reuben, *Everything You Always Wanted to Know About Sex.* (New York: Allen, 1970). Though certainly not written from a Christian viewpoint, this book has proved valuable in providing basic facts in an easily read fashion concerning sexuality in our society and other societies as well.

Middle Age and Aging

E. W. Busse and E. Pfeiffer, *Behavior and Adaptation in Late Life* (Boston: Little, Brown and Company, 1969). A good introduction to the life of the elderly from a scholarly point of view.

R. N. Butler and M. I. Lewis, *Aging and Mental Health* (Saint Louis: Mosby, 1973). The best brief introduction to aging and the emotional problems that occur with aging individuals.

Paul Tournier, *Learn to Grow Old* (New York: Harper and Row, 1972). A well-written but philosophical view of the Christian in late life.

Drug Abuse and Mental Retardation

American Medical Association, *Mental Retardation: A Handbook for Primary Physicians* (American Medical Association, 1965). Quite technical but a valuable introduction to mental retardation and a source book for references on counseling.

H. R. Greenberg, *What You Should Know About Drugs and Drug Abuse* (New York: School Book Services, 1971). An excellent and factual introduction to the different drugs that are being abused in our society.

Therapeutic Approaches

Behavior Therapy

Herbert Benson, *The Relaxation Response* (New York: Morrow, 1975). A good introduction to a classical type of the very popular relaxation therapies today. Benson works from a very sound scientific approach.

J. Wolpe, *The Practice of Behavior Therapy* (New York: Permagon Press, 1968). A somewhat technical but good introduction to behavior therapy.

Client-Centered Therapy

C. R. Rogers, *Client Centered Therapy* (Boston: Houghton Mifflin, 1951). The very popular client-centered approach to therapy is outlined.

Group Therapy

J. W. Knowles, *Group Counseling* (Englewood Cliffs, New Jersey: Prentice-Hall, 1964). A very good introduction to group dynamics and group therapy techniques by a pastoral counselor.

I. D. Yalom, *The Theory and Practice of Group Psychotherapy*

(New York: Basic Books, 1970). A technical but readable introduction to group therapy from a psychiatric point of view.

Logotherapy

V. Frankl, *Man's Search for Meaning* (New York: Washington Square Press, 1963). A popular approach to therapy that can easily be applied to the Christian orientation.

Marriage and Family Therapy

N. W. Ackerman, *The Psychodynamics of Family Life: Diagnosis and Treatment* (New York: Basic Books, 1958). The classical introduction by a very well-known family therapist.

V. Satir, *Conjoint Family Therapy* (Palo Alto, California: Science and Behavior Books, 1964). The classical introduction to Virginia Satir's family therapy model.

Psychoanalysis

S. Freud, *A General Introduction to Psychoanalysis* (New York: Liverright Publishing Corporation, 1920). The classic and best introduction to psychoanalysis in a very readable style.

Reality Therapy

W. Glasser, *Reality Therapy* (New York: Harper and Row, 1965). The classic introduction to a very popular type of therapy among Christian therapists.

Self-Concept Therapy

M. Maltz, *Psycho-Cybernetics* (Englewood Cliffs, New Jersey: Prentice-Hall, 1960). Probably the best introduction to the popular self-image and self-concept therapies being used today.

"Third Force" Therapies

F. Goble, *The Third Force* (New York: Pocket Books, 1971).

An introduction to the therapies and psychology of Abraham Maslow and other Third Force psychologists, such as Mowrer.

Transactional Analysis and Gestalt Therapy

T. A. Harris, *I'm OK: You're OK: A Practical Guide to Transactional Analysis* (New York: Harper and Row, 1967). The best introduction to transactional analysis in a very readable style.

Mental Health and Religion

J. E. Adams, *Competent to Counsel* (Grand Rapids: Baker Book House, 1970). A slanted and exceedingly narrow-minded view to counseling. However it does provide some useful scriptural basis for approaching certain types of problems.

G. Allport, *The Individual and His Religion* (New York: Mac-Millan, 1950). A good introduction to a theorist who considers psychology and religion extensively in his theoretical framework.

E. Fromm, *Psychoanalysis and Religion* (New York: Bantam, 1967). Of very little use to the Christian counselor, but it is a popular book the counselor should be acquainted with.

W. James, *The Varieties of the Religious Experience* (New York: New American Library, 1958). The classical work that introduced the subject of the relationship of psychology and religion into modern behavioral scientific thought.

K. Menninger, *Whatever Became of Sin?* (New York: Hawthorne, 1973). A very interesting view of sin from a classical psychoanalyst. It is very readable.

O. H. Mowrer, *The Crisis in Psychiatry and Religion* (New York: Van Nostrand, 1961). A very important view from a distinguished psychologist concerning guilt and the proper approach to guilt. Of great applicability to the Christian counselor.

E. F. Torrey, *The Mind Game: Witchdoctors and Psychiatrists* (New York: Emerson Hall, 1972). Though he does not discuss religion in particular, Torrey's sociological and anthropological views of psychiatry are very relevant to the relationship of psychiatry to religious healing.

Paul Tournier, *A Doctor's Casebook in Light of the Bible* (New York: Harper and Row, 1960). The application of a psychiatrist's practice in light of Christian principles.